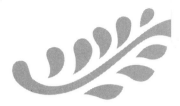

Aging and Vision Loss

A HANDBOOK FOR FAMILIES

Alberta L. Orr and Priscilla Rogers

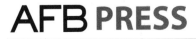

AFB PRESS

American Foundation for the Blind

Printed in the United States of America

Library of Congress Cataloging-in-Publication Data

Orr, Alberta L., 1950–
    Aging and vision loss : a handbook for families / Alberta L. Orr and
Priscilla Rogers.
        p.   cm.
    Includes bibliographical references.
    ISBN 0–89128–809–0 (pbk. : alk. paper)—ISBN 0–89128–810–4
(ASCII)
    1. Older people with visual disabilities—Care.   2. Vision disorders in
old age.   I. Rogers, Priscilla.   II. Title.
RE48.2.A5O733   2006
617.7'00846—dc22

                                                              2006011549

The American Foundation for the Blind—the organization to which Helen
Keller devoted her life—is a national nonprofit devoted to expanding the
possibilities for people with vision loss.

It is the policy of the American Foundation for the Blind to use in the first
printing of its books acid-free paper that meets the ANSI Z39.48 Standard.
The infinity symbol that appears above indicates that the paper in this
printing meets that standard.

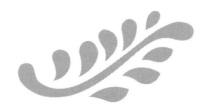

Contents

Preface

When you or someone you care about begins to experience vision loss, it may seem as though the world is going dark and life as you knew it is at an end. Although these feelings are understandable, finding that one's eyesight is diminished doesn't mean that one's life will be diminished as well.

If you have been searching for resources to help you understand and deal with a relative's vision loss, we hope you will find in this book, *Aging and Vision: Loss: A Handbook for Families*, answers to many of your questions and advice that meets many of your needs. Although we wrote *Aging and Vision* for readers who have a parent or older family member coping with the onset of age-related vision loss, it is designed to be useful to anyone trying to help someone who is having trouble with vision later in life.

Dealing with vision loss is not easy for anyone who may experience it, and an individual's loss of vision is often hard for family and friends as well. But today medical advances such as those relating to macular degeneration, up-to-date information on nutritional support of eyesight, and specialized products, technology, and adaptive techniques can help everyone make the most of their remaining vision. Through this book we hope to make a difference in the lives of millions of individuals by bringing hope, encouragement, and much-needed information.

Through this book, you will discover the service delivery system devoted to older people experiencing age-related vision loss.

You will also find a wealth of simple techniques for daily activities and independent living that will support adjustment, ongoing independence, and pursuit of life for the older person that you care about.

This handbook was written with you in mind, and it reflects the experiences, feelings, and concerns of people across the country who, along with their families, are trying to come to terms with a new awareness of visual impairment. We at the American Foundation for the Blind wish to thank them for sharing their experiences with us and you for allowing us the opportunity to reassure you and support you in turn.

Acknowledgments

The authors would like to acknowledge Ellen Bilofsky and Natalie Hilzen of AFB Press and Judy Scott of the AFB Center on Vision Loss for their efforts in making this book as factual and reader friendly as possible. Thanks also to Linda Harris and June Zeigler, family members, for reviewing the book and giving us their comments.

We would also like to thank the staff of the Center for the Visually Impaired in Atlanta, the Tennessee Services for the Blind and Visually Impaired in Nashville and Johnson City, and the Opportunity East Program of Lions Volunteer Blind Industries in Morristown, Tennessee for helping to set up focus groups with older people with vision loss and their family members; Kathy Gallagher from the National Industries for the Blind for conducting interviews; the staff from Title VII Chapter 2 Programs (Independent Living Services for Older Individuals Who Are Blind) in Alabama, Florida, Iowa, Missouri, Kansas, Mississippi, North Carolina, Oregon, Pennsylvania, Tennessee, and Utah for contributing interviews with older people with vision loss and with family members about their concerns, as well as materials about their programs for families; and Paige Berry, Deaf Blind Older Adult Specialist of the Helen Keller National Center for Deaf-Blind Youths and Adults for providing invaluable information on people with dual sensory loss.

We thank the following individuals in the Dallas area for allowing us to use their photographs in the book: Esther Smith and daughter Gwen Irwin; Donald V. Moore and son-in-law Frank Gay; Floy E. Dean, husband Wade Dean, and daughter Mary Ann Dean; Kay Weaver and daughter Annette W. Krell; Pat Higgins and orientation and mobility instructor Dave Jeppson; Claude Wood and daughter Joann Lawrence; Mary Castenada and son John Richard Navarro; Rae Burns, vision rehabilitation therapist; and Kay Hatcher and Kenneth Sawyer, employee of Tom Thumb Supermarket. Thanks also to Colonel Hugh Ketchum of Mississippi for allowing us to use his true story.

Introduction

MEET ROBERT MACKINNON

Robert Mackinnon, a 78-year-old widower, lives by himself six miles from town. He has always led an active life, and most sunny weekends you could find him golfing with friends, fly fishing on the lake, or tending his vegetable garden. Since his retirement from an auto insurance agency at the age of 65, he has been able to fish and golf during the week as well. After his wife passed away five years ago, Robert began cooking more as well, and he has found that he enjoys preparing meals for his friends and family when they visit.

Robert Mackinnon also has macular degeneration, a condition that caused him to lose the use of his central field of vision.

(Are you surprised? Keep reading.)

Although Robert had worn glasses for many years, three years ago he started noticing that he had difficulties writing checks, reading his mail, and telling time. His eyesight continued to deteriorate gradually, until he began to lose the ability to see things in the central field of his vision. Robert, a fiercely independent man who emigrated from Scotland 55 years ago, was reluctant to ask for help. Instead, he stopped doing the things that he loved one by one. For a while, his outlook was bleak.

Robert's daughter Sandra, who lives about 30 miles away, noticed the changes in her father. After watching him anxiously for several weeks, she realized that he was experiencing problems with his vision, and got him an appointment with an ophthalmologist. Robert was diagnosed as having a condition known as macular degeneration, which is fairly common among older people. Sandra found a local vision rehabilitation agency after contacting local hospitals, checking with her local librarian, and surfing the Internet to find organizations that provide services for people with vision loss. Then she spent some time negotiating with her father, with respect for his feelings and desire for independence, over the type of help he was willing to accept. Soon after, a professional called a vision rehabilitation therapist from the agency visited Robert at home and provided him with hands-on instruction about how to adjust to daily life with less sight. An orientation and mobility specialist taught him how to use a cane to get around his home and yard safely and how to make use of public transportation in his area. He learned a skill called eccentric viewing that helps him use his side vision to replace the central vision he has lost.

A year later, Robert Mackinnon takes care of his own daily needs. He still cooks, tends his garden, and—believe it or not—still plays golf. Through the local vision rehabilitation agency he found out about the United States Blind Golf Association, which offered encouragement, and he found a friend who was willing to coach him. He also enjoys reading with the help of free Talking Books on special cassette tapes. It wasn't easy getting here, but with the help of rehabilitation professionals, a vision loss support group, and in particular his daughter Sandra, Robert now knows that there is life after vision loss.

VISION LOSS—WHAT NOW?

Is someone in your family, like Robert, experiencing vision loss? Do you want to offer help, like Sandra, but are unsure about how to proceed? If so, you are not alone. As the population ages, more and more of our older relatives, friends, and neighbors are losing their vision to some degree. Although the wonders of modern medicine have extended our lives decades beyond what was the norm 100 years ago, the gift of longer life may be accompanied by certain eye conditions that are not a part of "normal" aging. Millions of people across the country are facing vision loss, either their own or that of elderly friends or relatives; and when an older person experiences vision loss, the entire family can be affected. The habits, roles, and relationships of a lifetime might need to be adjusted. Along with whatever feelings your older relative may be dealing with, you're probably experiencing a wide range of emotions yourself: fear, anxiety, grief, and anger. "Overwhelmed" is a word you may be finding yourself using more and more lately.

Don't lose hope.

Most people who lose some vision in their later years do not become totally blind. Although medicine hasn't solved every problem, eye conditions like cataracts and glaucoma can be managed successfully through outpatient surgery and intraocular lenses for cataracts and eye drops to control pressure for glaucoma; and research on others like macular degeneration may bring new advances as well. For people whose eyesight has become impaired, there are a wide variety of resources out there to help. A wealth of useful information has been gathered in this handbook, and it will show you how to utilize these resources, provide appropriate assistance to your loved one with vision loss, and understand the emotions that accompany these life changes. From coping with initial feelings of fear and loss to adapting a home for safe and independent living, the topics covered in this book are meant to provide you with the guidance and basic facts that you need. In the pages that fol-

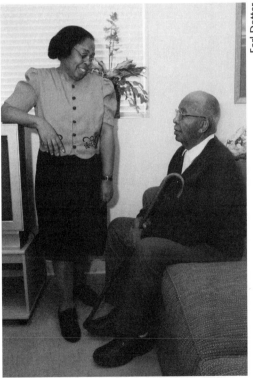

Earl Dotter

Although an older person's vision loss can affect the entire family, with good communication, understanding, and the right professional assistance, a successful adjustment is well within reach.

low, both practical information and supportive resources will be presented to help you and your relative successfully make the transition to life with vision loss.

This book opened at the end of the Mackinnon family's story in order to stress that however difficult the situation might seem to be at the moment, families can and do successfully make this transition. You'll meet other families throughout the book, each with their own specific concerns. Every family is different, but as you continue reading this handbook, you are likely to see some similarities between your own situation and the examples provided. The information and strategies provided in this book will help you and your older relative devise a plan that will work for you.

A PRELIMINARY NOTE

When an older family member experiences vision loss, family members and even friends commonly experience a variety of feelings, often beginning with fear and anxiety about their loved one's safety and well-being. But they are also frequently worried about the impact that this situation will have on their own lives. They may think they will have to become caregivers, giving up their freedom to devote at least part of their lives to be responsible for the safekeeping of someone who can no longer care for him- or herself. One of the primary goals of this book is to reassure you that your older relative does not need "caretaking" on the basis of vision loss alone. If your older relative who is experiencing vision loss does need some degree of care, it is likely that he or she has additional health or physical conditions, as many older people do.

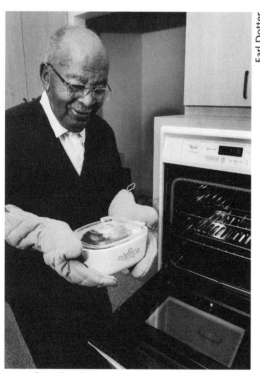

Earl Dotter

People who have lost some vision can still live independent lives. Your older relative does not need "caretaking" on the basis of vision loss alone.

If you are worried that your relative will always be needy and dependent, you will find that the chapters that follow will contradict that assumption. Instead of being a caregiver for your older relative, you can be someone who helps him or her to gather information, solve problems, and maintain progress. Probably more than anything else, your role will be to support and provide assistance to your older relative on his or her own journey.

OVERVIEW OF THIS HANDBOOK

Although this handbook is organized in a narrative format to follow the major stages of adjustment to vision loss, you may find that your family has already reached a later stage in the process. Maybe your mother has already been diagnosed with a particular vision loss condition and has begun to make the adjustments that will make life easier and more active. Or perhaps you simply want to figure out how to be a better advocate for your father with medical professionals. Readers can skip around this handbook to suit their family's specific needs. Here's what you'll find:

> *Chapter 1* contains an overview of how your family member will learn to cope with vision loss, and how you can help.

> *Chapter 2* presents basic facts about vision loss, including the difference between normal changes in the aging eye and more serious eye conditions, how to recognize signs of vision loss, and how to get information from eye care professionals.

> *Chapter 3* discusses the stages of adjustment to vision loss—including your own reactions as a family member.

> *Chapter 4* suggests ways to restore the equilibrium of family relationships through more effective communication and understanding of your relative's need to remain in control of his or her own life.

> *Chapter 5* describes services that are available to individuals with vision loss and how to find them.

Chapter 6 details specific new skills and helpful solutions for everyday tasks, such as cooking.

Chapter 7 outlines simple adaptations that can be made to make your relative's home safer and to make it easier to move around.

Chapter 8 offers information about dealing with vision loss along with other health conditions or disabilities, such as hearing impairment.

Chapter 9 discusses the support systems of family and friends that you and your relative may need.

Chapter 10 describes how people with vision loss can continue to enjoy and participate in leisure activities.

Frequently Asked Questions is a quick reference to common questions that you and your older relative may be wondering about.

Resources is a guide to organizations, information, products, and services that can be helpful to you and your relative.

Finally, remember as you begin to read that this book was written for *you,* to help with the emotions and difficult situations you may be experiencing since your older relative first began to lose vision and to give you the information you need to help your relative manage the adjustment to vision loss.

Chapter 1

Getting Started: The Basics

Sandra, Robert Mackinnon's daughter, had begun to suspect that her father might be losing his vision, although she wasn't sure. In the midst of all the overwhelming and frightening uncertainty, she was sure of only one thing: she loved her father. He could be cantankerous, opinionated, judgmental, and sometimes even downright exasperating—especially in the kitchen, where everything had to be done his way. But he was a wonderful father, and now a wonderful grandfather, and Sandra desperately wanted to do the right thing for him as he grew older and—seemingly for the first time in his life—needed some help.

But Sandra mostly had questions and no answers: "How can I help him? Will he even want my help? Is he actually losing his vision, or does he have some other problem? I live 30 miles away; will he need to move in with me? Will I have to give up my life and freedom to become a full-time caregiver for my father? How will that affect my marriage? My own children? My relationship with my father? Will my father be depressed for the rest of his life?" Sandra was concerned, and frightened, too.

What often scares us more than anything else is the unknown. When you begin to suspect that your parent or other older friend or relative is losing his or her vision, you might not have any idea where to begin to face the challenge. Like Sandra, you may feel lost in a whirlwind of questions—questions you're not even sure you want the answers to. The only thing you might be certain of is your desire to do what's best for your parent—yet you may wonder if that will be enough and how you will to know the right thing to do.

Before starting to answer all the questions you have, and even a few that you don't yet know to ask, let's lay the groundwork for the journey you and your family are about to embark upon. So sit back and take a deep breath. Let's talk about *you*.

THE EXPERIENCE OF VISION LOSS: WHAT YOU MIGHT BE THINKING

Vision loss does not have to result in a loss of independence, vitality, productivity, or activity. Nevertheless, many of us believe the opposite. We often imagine older people who are losing their vision as sitting sad and alone in the house, no longer engaging in the pastimes they once enjoyed. But your mother can not only engage in most, if not all, of her previous activities, she can even in all likelihood remain employed, if she has a job or wants to reenter the workforce. With the help of specialized devices designed for people who have vision loss, special vision rehabilitation services (such as training in accomplishing everyday tasks and using remaining vision), and a few simple tips for rearranging the house and its appliances, your father can live his life as before, without the assistance of full- or part-time help. There is also a range of resources and other services available to people who are visually impaired, and these will be discussed throughout this guide.

The trend in society today is toward providing services for older people that make it possible for them to remain in their own homes and familiar environments for as long as they can, with assistance only as needed. The value of staying within one's own home is very well established—both in terms of quality of life and expense. Although a visiting nurse, home health aide, or companion might be helpful for some people in some instances, if your older visually impaired relative does not have major health issues that require additional assistance, he or she most likely does not need "care" or a caregiver. In fact, taking on the role of caregiver might not be the best alternative for either you or your older relative. A more beneficial approach may be to focus on helping your older relative to function independently, maintain self-esteem, and remain a productive and vital part of the family and community. As you continue to read this book, you and your older relative will be able to make choices about what type of living environment is the best fit for your family.

MAKING IT WORK FOR *YOUR* FAMILY

Families are complicated. It is important to recognize that daughters, sons, siblings, and parents have all kinds of relationships with each other—both positive and negative. You may not get along with your father as well as Sandra does with hers; in fact, there might even be some real conflicts in your family's history. Some parents do not want help from their children and try to do everything for themselves, while others may expect a great deal of assistance and constant attention. Some people may always want to take responsibility for themselves and jump into work with a rehabilitation agency with gusto, while others want to be waited on rather than learning to do tasks independently. Others may shy away from the challenge of vision rehabilitation out of a fear that they will fail.

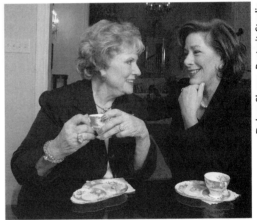

Debra Shore, Portrait Studio

Every family is unique. Finding out what your relative needs and wants is an important part of helping her make the choices that are right for her.

Every family is unique, and you will have to figure out how to apply the information and principles suggested here to your specific situation. Sandra, in the example that started this chapter, already knows that her father cherishes his independence. She'll need to take this into account as she tries to help him adjust to vision loss. You probably know your older relative well also. Consider what ideas and beliefs he or she holds as you begin to determine how to be helpful. Be prepared to listen to your relative's needs and wants and to really hear them. Examine your family's interpersonal dynamics to decide how you and the rest of your family can be most effective in helping your older relative. Most of all, remember that conflict within families during periods of change is normal. Most likely, you won't be able to avoid a little conflict, but you can be better prepared to resolve it.

Your family's own beliefs, values, culture, and traditions will no doubt come into play in the adjustment process. For example, some families are generally more comfortable receiving help from outside the family such as a home health aide, an occupational therapist, or a vision rehabilitation therapist (also known as a rehabilitation teacher) from a vision rehabilitation agency. Other people, however, feel they need to take the primary responsibility of caring for their own family members, or may rely more on neighbors, friends, their community, church, synagogue, or mosque than other families would. As a result, they may be less likely to seek outside help from a vision rehabilitation agency or respond to an offer of services. You and your family will be familiar with your own culture and traditions, of course, and communicating this information to the vision rehabilitation professionals with whom you'll work will also be a great help. For more resources on culture and diversity, take a look at the Resources section at the end of this book.

PAY ATTENTION TO YOURSELF, TOO

The suggestions in this book are based on the premise that it is best for everyone concerned if you look at yourself more as a helper rather than a caregiver with your older relative who is experiencing vision loss. But there's one person for whom you ought to remain a caregiver: *you*. Take good care of yourself. Helping your older relative adjust to vision loss may be challenging at times, and you will need to remember to give yourself breaks. Make sure that you set aside time in your life, no matter how busy you are, to simply relax and be good to yourself. Getting involved with a support group or even seeing a counselor can also help you with your own feelings and stress related to your older relative's vision loss and rehabilitation. Keep your own needs and emotions in mind as you try to be attentive to those of your relative.

Above all, remember that you don't have to solve every problem and face every challenge in the first day, week, or even

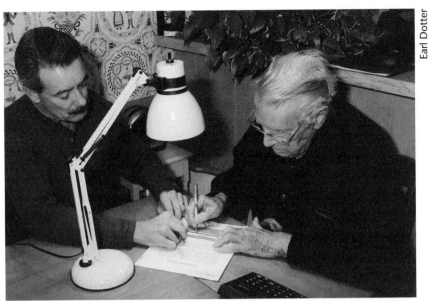

Adjustment takes time. You can solve problems—such as learning to sign a document using a signature guide—one at a time.

month. Helping your older relative adjust is a process that probably needs to be taken one step at a time. Although adjustment—any adjustment—can involve challenges, older people and their families *do* successfully adjust to vision loss—each in his or her own way and time frame. As you continue reading this book, keep in mind that your family will get there, too. Continue to imagine your own family's "success story." It might be a little hazy at first, but by the time you get to the end of this book, it will probably be a lot clearer.

FIRST STEPS

Beginning to learn about and adjust to vision loss in one's family can start with some basic information. Read through the list of first steps below, and keep these fundamental points in mind:

1. **Be aware of symptoms of vision loss** such as reports of sudden blurring in vision, double vision, flashes of lights, or halos around lights, or signs of vision loss such as reducing or stopping normal activities (leisure activities or reading, for example) or having problems getting around unfamiliar places. (More information about symptoms is covered in Chapter 2.)

2. **Understand the difference between normal changes in the eye** due to the aging process and the major causes of age-related vision loss. Some normal changes include the inability to focus at close range, decreased visual acuity, increased need for light, difficulty with glare, difficulty adapting to dark and light, and more trouble with contrast, depth perception, and colors. Many people also have increasing trouble from floaters and dry eyes. Everyone experiences these types of changes to one degree or another. In contrast, there are certain eye conditions that, although they are more common in older people, are not a normal part of aging and can lead to serious vision loss. These major age-related eye conditions include macular degeneration, glaucoma, diabetic retinopathy, and cataracts. (See Chapter 2 for more discussion of both normal changes and eye conditions.)

3. **Speak directly to your older relative experiencing vision loss about your concerns**, taking care to be sensitive as well as pragmatic. (Chapter 4 covers the topic of communication.)

4. **Recommend that your older relative see an eye care professional** as soon as possible if he or she is having symptoms of vision loss or has not seen an eye care professional in the last two years. Some—but not all—eye conditions may be progressive (gradually becoming worse); some have more options for treatment than others. It is important to determine what can be done to make the best use of the vision remaining. There are two types of eye care professionals: ophthalmologists and optometrists. *Ophthalmologists* are medical doctors with a specialization in the functioning of the eye and eye diseases. They can diagnose eye conditions and perform eye surgery. *Optometrists* are not medical doctors, but they are eye care specialists and can diagnosis and treat eye conditions without surgery. Start with the ophthalmologist, if possible, to diagnose any eye condition.

5. **Ask for a referral to a low vision specialist.** Most of the age-related eye conditions that older people develop do not result in total blindness. A *low vision specialist* is an eye care professional who can help your older relative make the best use of his or her remaining vision. Ophthalmologists and (more

often) optometrists may have this specialization. Your eye care provider (assuming he or she is not a low vision specialist), can provide you with a referral to a low vision specialist for a low vision evaluation—although you might need to ask specifically for this referral. (If your eye care specialist is unable to provide a referral, contact

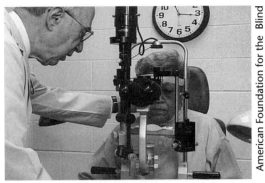

An eye exam by a low vision specialist is the first step in learning how to make the best use of an individual's existing vision.

the American Foundation for the Blind [AFB] or consult the service finder on AFB's Web site [www.afb.org] for a low vision center or referral source for low vision services in your area.) The low vision specialist uses special low vision eye charts to determine the level of vision and to prescribe low vision devices that may help, and he or she can teach your older relative how to use these assistive optical devices that can make reading and other close-up or distance tasks possible.

6. **Find out about local vision rehabilitation services.** Most older people who are experiencing age-related vision loss can learn to do many routine daily activities for themselves. Specialized agencies (frequently referred to as vision rehabilitation agencies or agencies for the blind and visually impaired), provide training and services to help them learn new adaptive techniques that will allow them to begin to feel independent again. Specialized vision-related services are available in every state, although there may be waiting lists in some locations. Depending upon where you live, an agency may be right in your local community; in rural areas, an agency may be farther away. Although information about services and specialized providers will be described in more detail in Chapter 6, some suggestions for how to begin are offered here in "Getting Help: Where to Start."

These services are provided by specially trained professionals, and as a family member you can help reinforce these new skills yourself. Many vision rehabilitation agencies involve family members in the older person's vision rehabilitation sessions so the family member can see firsthand the kinds of skills being taught, how the older person can be safe doing these activities by using these techniques, and how to be supportive.

7. **Do-It-Yourself.** Some techniques that can be used to continue everyday activities can be learned on your own, such as signing one's name using a writing guide, reading large-print materials, or using an alarm clock with large numerals. You can also start to look around the house for ways of making it easier and safer to get around. (See Chapters 6 and 7 for more information.)

GETTING HELP: WHERE TO START

Older people who are experiencing vision loss and their families need to know about the various types of agencies that provide services at both the state and local levels. Many of these are government agencies that provide services based on eligibility criteria, such as age or a certain degree of vision loss, but there are also private nonprofit vision rehabilitation agencies or low vision centers that may have exactly the type of services your older relative needs.

A quick way to find many of these services in your state is through the directory published by the American Foundation for the Blind, the *AFB Directory of Services for Blind and Visually Impaired Persons in the United States and Canada* (see the Resources section), which lists contacts for state aging and rehabilitation agencies, as well as local agencies that provide various types of vision services within each state. A free online search of this directory is available at www.afb.org/services.asp. You can also contact AFB's information help line, (800) 232-5463, or one of the other national organizations listed in the Resources section. More detailed information about the following types of services and how they can help your older relative appears in Chapter 5.

Vision Rehabilitation Services

When looking for vision-related services, you would probably want to start with the state rehabilitation agency, which will offer comprehensive services based on its assessment of an individual's needs. Offerings from private agencies will vary. If your relative is a veteran of U.S. military service, he or she will also be eligible for rehabilitation services from the Department of Veterans Affairs.

State vocational rehabilitation agencies: These agencies provide or fund specific rehabilitation services. In some states there is a separate state agency that provides services just for people who are blind or visually impaired. In either case, the agency would offer the following vision rehabilitation services, which are described in more detail in Chapter 5:

- counseling
- independent living services—instruction provided by a vision rehabilitation therapist in how to carry out everyday tasks and get around indoors
- orientation and mobility instruction—instruction in traveling safely and independently, indoors and outdoors
- low vision services—prescription of special low vision devices to help make the best use of remaining vision and training in the use of these devices
- vocational services

Private agencies for people who are blind or visually impaired: Local, usually nonprofit agencies, that provide vision rehabilitation services. They may do so privately and/or under contract with state rehabilitation agencies.

Low vision clinics: Separate clinics that provide special examinations for people with low vision, low vision devices, and training in how to use the devices

Aging Network Services

You may also be interested in services provided specifically for older persons. The U.S. Administration on Aging administers a network of Area Agencies on Aging that can then link the individual to local services, such as Meals on Wheels, transportation, senior centers, and congregate dining. The easiest way to get such referrals is from the Eldercare Locator toll-free number (800) 677-1116 or Web site www.eldercare.gov. State contact information for aging services also appears in the *AFB Directory of Services.*

(*continued on next page*)

GETTING HELP (*continued*)

Other Types of Assistance

Supplemental Security Income: The Supplemental Security Income (SSI) program provides assistance to individuals with limited income and resources or disabilities. To qualify for SSI, a person must be age 65 or older or legally blind or disabled (that is, unable to work because of physical or mental problems), and have income below a specified level. It is administered by the Social Security Administration, the federal agency that also administers Social Security. Information about SSI is available from the Social Security Administration toll-free number (800) 772-1213 or its Web site www.ssa.gov.

Medicaid: Medicaid is a state-administered program that helps to pay the costs of medical care, hospitalization, and nursing home care for people whose income and resources fall below a certain level. Generally, those who are eligible for SSI are also eligible for Medicaid. Information about Medicaid is available from your local department of social services, whose listing generally can be found in the telephone book white pages under the state or county listings. This department will also offer information about other services, such as food stamps.

HELPING FROM A DISTANCE

Not everyone lives as close to his or her older relatives as Sandra does to her father. Many adult children and other relatives are faced with the challenge of providing assistance to their older relative from hundreds of miles away, or even from another part of the country entirely. Although more effort and persistence may be required to construct a plan that will enable your older relative to live at home and continue to function independently, it can be done. If finances permit, you might want to hire a gerontologist, geriatric social worker, or case manager who is in your area to work with your older relative to develop a plan and to locate nearby services and resources (see "Finding Help from a Distance"). If this is not an option, you can help your parent or other older relative contact the state rehabilitation agency and the local aging organization called the Area Agency on Aging for a referral.

FINDING HELP FROM A DISTANCE

While geriatric care managers are frequently licensed by the state within their respective fields of expertise, there are no state or national regulations for professional care managers. For this reason, anyone can use the title case or care manager. However, membership in a professional organization or certification in care management are good indicators of appropriate background. One such organization is the National Association of Professional Geriatric Care Managers (see the Resources Section for more information), which provides a search for members, by zip code, on its Web site (www.caremanager.org).

There are many resources available online to help and provide information. A connection with a reputable organization is an indicator of reliability. Other sources for referrals include:

- your local Area Agency on Aging (call (800) 677-1116 or go to www. eldercare.gov for the agency in your area)
- local hospitals and health maintenance organizations
- geriatricians
- senior or family service organizations
- senior centers
- religious organizations, including churches, synagogues, and mosques
- telephone book listings for Senior Citizens' Services, Care Management, Home Care, Home Health Services, and similar subject areas
- Medicaid offices
- private care management companies

Now you know that help is available for older people who are losing their vision and their families. But, you may not even be sure whether vision loss is really the source of your relative's problems. The next chapter discusses how to recognize the signs of vision loss and what to do about them, as well as explaining the difference between the typical changes in vision that affect people as they get older and potentially serious eye conditions.

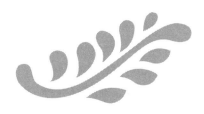

Chapter 2

Recognizing the Signs of Vision Loss

Dad knocked his knee—hard—on the coffee table again this week when I was visiting," noted Sandra McIntosh to her sister, Carrie, over the phone. "God only knows what accidents he might have when I'm not around. He's really taking it slow on the stairs, too."

"Well, he's not young anymore. That's probably typical for someone his age," Carrie replied.

"No, I don't think so. It wasn't two months ago that Dad was out golfing every Saturday."

"You know, come to think of it, a couple of weeks ago when I took the kids by for a visit," remembered Carrie, "he didn't enjoy cooking for us the way he usually does. He was squinting at the cookbook, and he had the heat on the oven up way too high. He burned lunch, and we had to eat out. I don't ever remember Dad burning anything before."

"Do you think there's something wrong with his eyes?" asked Sandra.

"I really don't know. Are those the signs?"

It's not always obvious to others that someone is experiencing vision loss. Many older people are too proud or afraid to admit that they are having problems seeing, and their loved ones might not know what to make of the subtle changes in behavior that can accompany vision loss. Sometimes, changes in vision happen so slowly that the person himself or herself doesn't realize that a problem may be developing and attributes them to "just getting older, I guess." On occasion, signs of vision loss can even be mistaken for early signs of dementia! The variety of possible eye conditions complicates matters even further, since they can present many different symptoms. Some changes in the eyes of older people are normal and do not indicate a serious condition. But others point to the possibility of something potentially serious.

Like Sandra and her sister, you might not be sure if your older relative is experiencing vision loss at all. This chapter is designed to present you with the facts about vision loss: what is normal, what is not, and how to recognize the difference.

NORMAL CHANGES IN THE AGING EYE

It is helpful to understand that normal changes occur in our eyes as we age, and these may affect functioning to some degree day by day. "Normal" means that the changes occur almost universally among people as they age and are no cause for alarm, although they may require some getting used to. What follows are detailed descriptions of nine normal changes in the aging eye to help you and your older relative understand how vision may change with age. Remember, however, that everyone's eyes need to be checked regularly, and if you have any concerns about the nature of vision problems your older relative is experiencing, he or she should see an eye care professional as soon as possible. (See "Tips for Eye Protection.")

PRESBYOPIA

Presbyopia will be familiar to you if you are over 40 or know someone who is. When you begin to hold your reading material further and further away to keep it in focus, you are experiencing presbyopia. With age, the muscles of the eye that allow us to focus at close distances gradually become less elastic. Most older people cannot focus comfortably at an average 16-inch reading distance and have difficulty reading small print, like newspapers or labels on medicine bottles, for instance. Presbyopia occurs

TIPS FOR EYE PROTECTION

- Have an annual comprehensive eye exam that includes dilation of the pupils by an eye care professional. People over 50 should do this yearly.

- People diagnosed with a particular eye condition need to have an on-going relationship with a physician who is a specialist in that condition and consult regularly with him or her. Topics to discuss include any changes in vision, medications, and activities that should be avoided.

- Be aware of the signs of vision loss and contact your eye care professional right away if you or your relative experiences any of them.

- Support eyes with good nutrition. Recent research indicates that vitamins such as those found in leafy green vegetables, including antioxidants, zinc, and lutein, help to maintain good eye health and to prevent conditions such as macular degeneration.

- Protect eyes from glare and wear UVA/UVB–protective sunglasses to help prevent or slow development of cataracts. Avoid overexposure to sun.

- Wear protective eye gear for certain sports, close crafts, and work activities when necessary to prevent injuries.

- Try to maintain a healthy lifestyle, including avoiding smoking and engaging in exercise to prevent obesity, which can raise blood pressure and pressure in the eye.

normally and is correctable with bifocals, reading glasses, or contact lenses.

REDUCED VISUAL ACUITY

You may be aware that the normal *visual acuity* (see "Terms Describing Vision Loss" later in this chapter) for a younger person is 20/20. The normal acuity for an older person, however, is 20/40, just slightly reduced from 20/20. An acuity of 20/40 means that, normally, older people are expected to see at a 20-foot distance what a younger person with 20/20 vision sees at

40 feet away. This is not a dramatic reduction for the aging person who can see well enough to function normally and continue driving.

INCREASED NEED FOR LIGHT

Your parent or other older relative may seem to have an *increased need for light.* You may notice that your older relative is trying to sit directly under the lamplight in order to try to read something, or may be using higher wattage light bulbs. This is common.

As people grow older, the smaller pupil and increased haziness of the lens of the eye cause less light to reach the back of the eye. Although the normal lens of a younger person's eye is clear and allows light through it, the center of the lens in an older person turns yellow and loses the ability to focus on close tasks, such as reading or doing a handcraft. Eventually the lens turns an amber color and then brown, letting in less and less light. An older person requires *four times* more light than a younger person—by 80 years of age perhaps *ten times* more light.

You may want to suggest that your older relative increase the wattage of light bulbs around the house. Dispensing light more evenly throughout the room with more lamps might help as well. Natural sunlight is generally the best lighting for reading or close work, and natural sunlight bulbs, which emit the same type of white light as sunlight, are now available commercially. (See the Resources section at end of this book for information about lighting.)

DIFFICULTY ADAPTING TO LIGHT AND DARK

Decreased ability to *adapt to light and dark* environments is something we can all understand. When you go into a movie theater, it may take you a while to adjust from the light to be able to see in the dark. This adjustment can take an older person as long as 20 minutes, and adjusting from a dark environment to a light environment, which is not as difficult, can take up to 7 or 8 minutes.

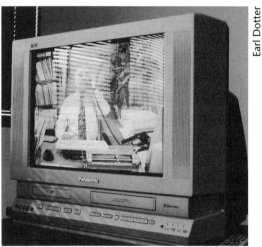

Earl Dotter

The glare on this television screen makes it difficult to see.

DIFFICULTY WITH GLARE

The ability to recover from *glare* begins to decrease around age 50. Glare results when bright light enters the eye, either directly or through reflection. Glass table-tops, polished wooden floors, mirrors, and TV screens are the usual sources of glare. Glossy paint can also be a problem, and glare from glossy paper, such as that used in a magazine, can make print hard to read. Your older relative might want to take this into consideration in organizing his or her living space. (See Chapter 7 for suggestions.)

REDUCED CONTRAST SENSITIVITY

Contrast sensitivity refers to the ability to detect differences between light and dark areas. For example, if a room in your mother's home had white walls, a white door frame, and white door, she might have difficulty locating the room's exit. Painting the doorframe a dark contrasting color would help her see the door. The same principle would apply to printed materials. A book cover with a background of royal blue and white print is much easier to read than is black print on the blue background. (How to evaluate and modify a home environment to make it easier to get around is discussed in greater detail in Chapter 7.)

REDUCED ABILITY TO SEE COLORS

The ability to see *color* also diminishes with age. Deeper, saturated colors such as red and royal blue are much easier to see than pastels. Solid colors are also easier to see than patterns.

REDUCED ABILITY TO SEE DEPTH

You may notice that your older relative hesitates at the top of a flight of stairs or on a sidewalk curb. Since *depth perception* decreases with age, older people may have difficulty seeing clearly where the stairs or the curb begins. Loss of depth perception, although normal, is a serious matter, since trips and falls can result. In fact, vision loss is one of the largest contributors to falls that can result in serious injury among the older population. Placing brightly colored tape or paint—bright orange or yellow works best—at the edge of each step in his or her home will help your older relative see where each step begins.

FLOATERS AND DRY EYES

Floaters are tiny spots or specks that float across the field of vision. Most people notice them in well-lit rooms or outdoors in the bright sunlight. Usually, floaters are harmless. If bright flashes of light surround the floaters, however, this may indicate a more serious problem. If your parent or older relative is seeing flashes of light of any kind, consult an eye care professional as soon as possible.

Dry eyes result when the aging eye is no longer able to produce tears in the way it does in younger people. Dry eyes can be irritating but can usually be remedied by using eye drops made for this purpose.

HINTS OF SOMETHING MORE SERIOUS

Although the changes in vision just described are experienced by just about everyone, certain changes can signal that something unusual or serious is taking place. Some signs of vision change can indicate that there is a need to be evaluated as soon as possible by an eye care professional, either an ophthalmologist or optometrist.

IF YOUR OLDER RELATIVE describes any of the following symptoms to you, explain to him or her that these can be signs of a serious vision problem and that it is important to get to an eye care professional immediately.

- Sudden hazy or blurred vision
- Recurrent pain in or around the eye
- Double vision
- Seeing flashes of light
- Seeing halos around lights
- Unusual sensitivity to light or glare
- Changes in the color of the iris
- Sudden development of persisting floaters

COMMON EYE CONDITIONS

In contrast to the normal vision changes that affect virtually all people as they get older, certain conditions that affect many older adults can cause serious vision loss. But how would you know if your older relative is beginning to lose some vision? What if he or she doesn't tell you about problems he or she is having, out of fear, pride, or some other reason? There are still ways to tell, by watching for the following observable signs.

SIGNS OF VISION LOSS

Exhibiting the following behaviors, among others, in any of these areas, may be indicative of vision loss:

Moving around the Environment
- Constantly bumping into objects
- Having difficulty walking on irregular or bumpy surfaces
- Stepping hesitantly
- Going up and down stairs slowly and cautiously
- Shuffling feet
- Brushing against the wall while walking
- Missing objects by under-reaching or over-reaching

Performing Everyday Activities
- Changing the way one reads, watches television, drives, walks, or engages in hobbies—or discontinuing one or more of these activities
- Squinting or tilting the head to the side in order to focus on an object
- Indicating difficulty in identifying faces or objects
- Demonstrating problems locating personal objects even in a familiar environment
- Reaching out for objects in an uncertain manner
- Having trouble identifying colors; selecting clothing in unusual combinations of colors or patterns

Eating and Drinking
- Demonstrating problems getting food onto a fork
- Having difficulty cutting food or serving from a serving dish
- Spilling food off the plate while eating
- Pouring liquids over the top of a cup or drinking glass
- Knocking over liquids while reaching across the table for another item

Reading and Writing
- Ceasing to read mail, newspapers, or books
- Holding reading material very close to the face or at an angle
- Writing less clearly than previously and showing difficulty writing on a line
- Finding lighting in a room inadequate for reading and other activities

Sometimes, however, the behaviors just listed may indicate confusion as well. It is important to determine whether your older relative is exhibiting symptoms of a vision problem or some other condition, such as dementia. If you're not sure, then you might want to consult with an internist or family physician, as well as an eye care professional.

If you and your older relative are concerned that the symptoms he or she experiences are beyond those normally associated with the aging eye, you both probably want to know what sorts of conditions might be involved. The four leading eye conditions associated with aging are *macular degeneration, diabetic retinopathy, glaucoma,* and complicated *cataracts.* Sometimes, older individuals can experience more than just one of these conditions. What follows is a brief outline of all of these eye conditions, designed to serve as a background for your trip to an eye care professional and to provide basic helpful information. And, since eye care professionals may use terms with specialized meanings to describe your relative's vision loss, some of them are explained in "Terms Describing Vision Loss."

TERMS DESCRIBING VISION LOSS

Visual acuity is the sharpness of vision with respect to the ability to distinguish detail. It is often measured by the eye's ability to distinguish details and shapes of objects at a given distance. In the United States it is usually expressed in a form such as 20/200, which means that the individual with this acuity can see at 20 feet what someone with 20/20, or normal vision, can see at 200 feet.

Legal blindness is a legal term used in the United States to determine eligibility for many types of government benefits and services, so it's important to know if this term applies to your older relative. Legal blindness is defined as a visual impairment in which distance visual acuity is 20/200 or less in the better eye after best correction with conventional lenses like eyeglasses or contact lenses (see *visual acuity*), or in which the individual has a visual field restriction of 20 degrees or less. An individual's full visual field is approximately 175–180 degrees, so a visual field of only 20 degrees is quite limited (see *visual field*).

Low vision means that a person who is visually impaired has vision loss even with regular corrective eyeglasses or contact lenses, but still has some useable vision and can learn to make the best use of it. People with low vision can use their available vision to perform daily tasks, with or without optical or nonoptical devices (see Chapter 8).

Visual field loss indicates some impairment in the field of vision. The field of vision is the area you see when looking straight ahead. If you try to

MACULAR DEGENERATION

Macular degeneration is the leading cause of vision loss among older people and occurs most frequently among Caucasians. Macular degeneration weakens the macula, the center portion of the eye responsible for central vision and that is needed to see detail. This condition results in blurred vision in the center of the eye and can also cause blind spots in the center of vision.

There are two types of macular degeneration, the wet type and the dry type. The dry type is more common and less severe and typically comes on gradually. It is caused by atrophy or thinning of the macula's tissue. The wet condition usually occurs quickly, so you and your older relative should see an eye care professional for immediate treatment if you recognize its

TERMS DESCRIBING VISION LOSS *(continued)*

look straight ahead, you will notice that you can see much more than what is directly in front of you. In fact, you can see nearly a semicircle, approximately 175 to 180 degrees. Some types of vision loss cause loss of vision only in certain parts of the visual field. Vision field loss generally falls into three types: loss of central vision, loss of peripheral vision, and overall blurring.

- *Loss of central vision* refers to a loss of vision in the middle of your visual field. Central field loss makes it difficult to read, see a photograph, do other close-up tasks, and recognize faces. This type of vision loss would typically result if your older relative had macular degeneration.

- *Loss of peripheral vision* refers to the loss of side vision that can make it difficult to move about the environment with ease and safety. Glaucoma is one eye condition that results in peripheral field loss and can result in tunnel vision. A person with tunnel vision sees only what could be seen when looking through a narrow tube.

- *Overall blurring* means that the entire visual field is distorted. This is the type of field loss typically involved with cataracts. Diabetic retinopathy can also cause overall blurring coupled with spots of darkness in the visual field.

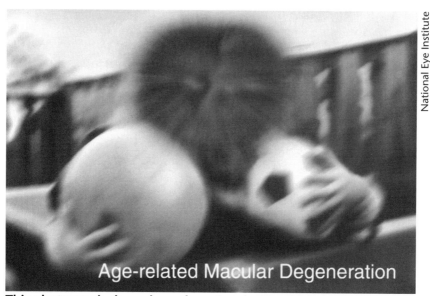

Age-related Macular Degeneration

This photograph shows how these two boys might appear to a person with macular degeneration, which leaves a blind spot in the middle of the visual field.

onset. The wet form is called wet because in its advanced stages it causes rapid growth of the small blood vessels beneath the retina. The affected blood vessels leak blood and other fluid, which form scar tissue. The result is a more severe vision loss.

IF YOUR OLDER RELATIVE has macular degeneration, he or she might experience:
- Blurry areas on a printed page
- Straight lines appearing wavy or bent
- Dark, empty spaces in the center of his or her vision

Macular degeneration is a serious condition, but it does not in itself result in total blindness. A low vision specialist can help an older person learn to use side vision—called *eccentric viewing*—for reading and other tasks for which central vision is ordinarily used. Once this skill is mastered, it can make a big dif-

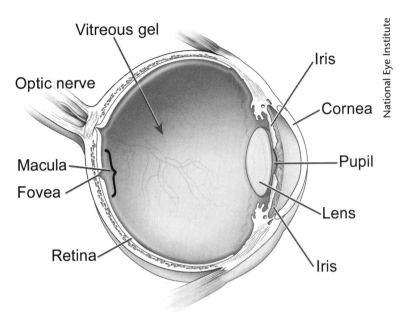

National Eye Institute

Macular degeneration affects the portion of the retina, called the macula, which controls detailed vision in the center of the visual field.

ference in what your older relative can see and how he or she can function.

GLAUCOMA

Glaucoma is caused by an increased level of pressure in the eye, referred to as intraocular pressure, caused by the buildup of excess fluid. The result is a loss of peripheral or side vision, which mostly affects older people's mobility, or their ability to move around safely in the environment. This loss of visual field can affect reading as well, since only a few words or letters may be seen at one time.

If not detected and treated, chronic elevated pressure in the eye can cause damage to the optic nerve, the bundle of nerve fibers that carries images to the brain. Once there is damage to the optic nerve, nothing can be done to reverse this condition. Glaucoma is dangerous because it can develop without symptoms. Often vision loss occurs without the person being aware at first. Because of this lack of symptoms, it is sometimes referred to as "the sneak thief of sight," and for all these reasons, an annual eye checkup with a glaucoma test is recommended for everyone.

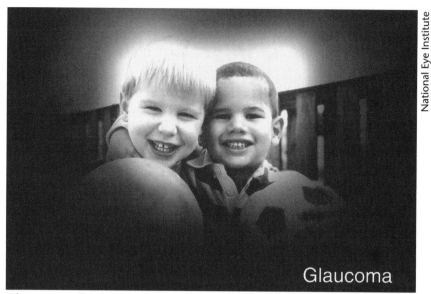

Glaucoma

Glaucoma affects peripheral, or side, vision, causing a tunnel vision effect.

There are two types of glaucoma: open angle and closed angle. Open-angle glaucoma occurs when the eye's drainage canals gradually become clogged, and this form of glaucoma is slow to affect vision. Closed-angle glaucoma results from blockage of the angle formed between two parts of the eye, the iris and the cornea, where fluid normally drains. It usually has a sudden or acute onset and is characterized by blurred vision, nausea, headache, and seeing halos around bright light. If your older relative experiences these symptoms, he or she should visit an ophthalmologist immediately. African Americans and Latinos are at a higher risk of developing glaucoma than are Caucasians, sometimes as early as age 40, and should have glaucoma checks beginning at age 35–40.

IF YOUR OLDER RELATIVE has closed-angle glaucoma, he or she might experience:
- Blurred vision
- Nausea
- Headache
- Seeing halos around bright lights

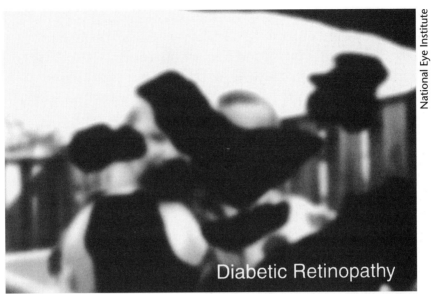

National Eye Institute

Diabetic Retinopathy

Diabetic retinopathy causes scattered blind spots, overall blurring, and loss of side vision that can vary from day to day.

DIABETIC RETINOPATHY

Diabetic retinopathy is associated with diabetes and can also cause cataracts and glaucoma. It occurs when diabetes damages the tiny blood vessels inside the retina—the light-sensitive tissue at the back of the eye. Blood vessels may leak fluid, causing damage that will lead to overall blurring or blind spots.

All people with diabetes, both Type 1 and Type 2, are at risk of developing this condition. Between 40 to 45 percent of Americans diagnosed with diabetes have some stage of diabetic retinopathy. In addition, older people who are African American, Latino, or Native American have a greater risk of developing diabetic retinopathy.

Some studies show that better control of blood sugar levels slows the onset and progression of diabetic retinopathy. A landmark study completed in 1993, known as the Diabetes Control and Complications Trial, and supported by more recent follow-ups, indicated that a strict regimen of blood sugar control reduced the risk for developing retinopathy by 76 percent. The strict regimen (involving a number of daily blood sugar tests, and use of an insulin pump or at least three insulin injections per day) also slowed the progression of the disease for people who had already developed some eye damage, and reduced the risk of kidney damage, nerve damage, heart problems, and stroke as well.[1] This degree of blood sugar control may not be best for everyone, however, including some older persons and people with heart disease, so it is important to consult with a physician before attempting it.

In addition to maintaining control of blood sugar levels, everyone with diabetes should have a comprehensive eye exam at least once a year in which the pupils are dilated with eye drops to allow the eye care professional to better see inside the eye. People with proliferative retinopathy (an advanced stage in which fragile new blood vessels grow that can break or leak) can reduce their risk of blindness significantly with timely treatment and appropriate follow-up care.

People with diabetic retinopathy often don't experience any symptoms until the condition has already become serious. Because the disease can progress without symptoms, annual dilated eye examinations for people with diabetes are crucial.

IF YOUR OLDER RELATIVE has diabetic retinopathy, he or she might experience:
- Blurred vision
- Blind spots as a result of bleeding in the eye

COMPLICATED CATARACTS

A cataract is a cloudy area that forms in the lens of the eye, affecting vision. Most cataracts form slowly and cause no pain, redness, or tearing of the eye. They can usually be treated successfully by surgery on an outpatient basis with a 95 percent success rate. However, in some cases, cataract extraction is not possible because of the potential for complications due to other eye conditions, lack of vision in the other eye, or other health concerns. For example, cataracts may be associated with diabetes. Older people who have cataracts tend to shield their eyes from bright light and glare and usually report that their vision is becoming hazier and hazier.

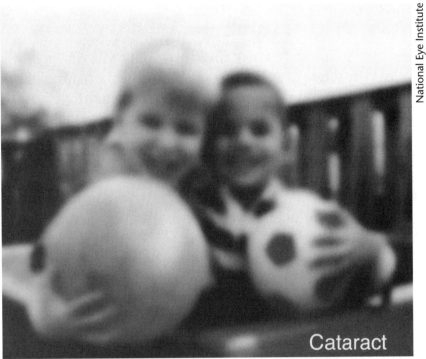

Cataract

National Eye Institute

Cataracts cause an overall blurring and haziness of vision

IF YOUR OLDER RELATIVE has complicated cataracts, he or she might experience:
- Reduced acuity
- Blurriness throughout the entire visual field
- Poor contrast sensitivity
- Sensitivity to light

OTHER CONDITIONS OF NOTE

In addition to the four leading eye conditions just discussed, there are two other conditions that are important to mention, although they are not themselves eye conditions. These are *hemianopia* and *Charles Bonnet Syndrome.*

HEMIANOPIA AND OTHER VISUAL COMPLICATIONS OF STROKE

A stroke can sometimes affect an individual's vision. The type of vision loss caused by a stroke depends on the area of the brain affected: there may be little or no visual impairment, or any combination of poor visual acuity, visual field loss, double vision, distortion, glare sensitivity, and visual perceptual difficulties.

Hemianopia is the loss of vision in half the visual field as the result of a cerebral stroke, or possibly a brain tumor or trauma. The most common defect, right homonymous hemianopia, occurs in the right half of the field of vision in both eyes. Hemaniopia can also occur in the corresponding halves of the left field of vision (*left homonymous hemianopia*), in the upper half of the field (*superior hemianopia*), the lower half (*inferior hemianopia*), or both outer halves of the field (*bitemporal hemianopia*).

Hemianopia interferes with reading because it makes it difficult for the person to find the next line of print. Also, the individual may consistently bump into objects on the affected side. The older person in such cases needs to make use of his or her remaining vision, and this can take some time and work with rehabilitation professionals. A low vision specialist may prescribe prism lenses, which bend incoming light to expand the field of vision.

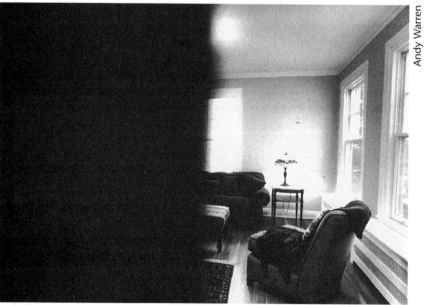

Andy Warren

Hemianopia as a result of a stroke distorts or eliminates vision in half the visual field.

IF YOUR OLDER RELATIVE has hemianopia following a stroke, he or she might experience:
- Loss of vision in half the visual field
- Decreased night vision
- Need for more light

CHARLES BONNET SYNDROME

Charles Bonnet Syndrome (CBS) is a little-known manifestation of vision loss that is experienced by some people with visual impairment. It consists of visual hallucinations that can seem quite real. People with CBS may see hallucinations of patterns and lines, which can become quite intricate, resembling brickwork, mosaic, or tiles. They may also see more complicated images of people, places, landscapes, and groups of people—sometimes life size and other times in miniature. These images appear out of the blue and can continue for a few minutes or sometimes several hours. Although CBS can affect people of any age, the condition usually only affects people who have lost their sight later in life. Despite the fact that the syndrome is not well known, it affects from 10 to 40 percent of people with low vision.[2] The hallucinations usually occur after a period of decreasing vision and when the person is alone or in bed at night, and often cease altogether within a year to 18 months. At present, there is no cure for CBS.

Sometimes the complicated images can make it difficult to get around. For example, a street or room may seem to take on a different shape, making it difficult to navigate. One individual described how, on approaching the top of a staircase, he had a vision of being on top of a mountain. Needless to say, he had difficulty getting down the stairs! Good knowledge of one's immediate surroundings can help overcome problems caused by hallucinations associated with CBS. Sometimes turning a light on and off or changing one's position from sitting to standing can help. Although there is no designated treatment for CBS, people who experience these symptoms can talk to their eye care professional to learn more about their condition.

Although the condition has been noted for many years, it rarely comes to the attention of many medical professionals, possibly because people experiencing CBS seldom talk about their experiences out of fear of being diagnosed with a mental illness. While hallucinations can be a sign of a sign of mental illness, however, CBS is strictly a result of vision loss. Once people understand the source of the images, they generally do not find them disturbing.

GATHERING FURTHER INFORMATION

Once your older relative receives an official diagnosis of a particular eye condition, you might want to expand your knowledge about his or her eye condition. An excellent source for more information about eye conditions, low vision, and the latest research is the National Eye Institute (NEI) of the National Institutes of Health. Its Web site is at www.nei.nih.gov. NEI also has many publications available. The Resources section at the end of this book gives contact information for NEI and other sources of information. In addition, it is important to speak to your relative's ophthalmologist or other eye care professional to understand his or her situation and to establish a good working relationship.

TALKING TO THE DOCTOR

With the basic information offered here about different age-related eye conditions, you have a good foundation for asking questions when you and your older relative visit a physician or an eye care specialist. Help your relative prepare for the visit by making a list of topics and questions he or she wants to discuss. As with most visits to a physician, it is usually helpful for an older person to have someone go along with him or her to ask questions and record information.

Today, patients take an active role in their health care. Your older relative, his or her physician, and you will be partners in the effort to achieve the best possible level of vision and quality of life for your older relative. An important part of this relationship is good communication. The questions in the accompanying list are important ones for you and your older relative to ask the physician or eye care specialist to get the discussion started.

QUESTIONS FOR THE EYE CARE PROFESSIONAL

The following questions highlight information that you and your older relative will want to obtain from the eye care professional. Since it is often difficult for the person being examined to focus on everything the doctor is saying, you should be prepared to help your older relative ask these questions.

About the Disease or Disorder . . .

- What is the diagnosis?
- What caused the condition?
- Can the condition be treated?
- How will this condition affect my vision now and in the future?
- Should we watch for any particular symptoms and notify you if they occur?
- Should I make any lifestyle changes?
- How often should I see you or any other eye care professional?

About Treatment . . .

- What is the treatment for the condition?
- When will the treatment start, and how long will it last?
- What are the benefits of this treatment, and how successful is it?
- What are the risks and side effects associated with this treatment?
- Are there foods, drugs, or activities that should be avoided with this treatment?
- If the treatment includes taking a medication, what should I do if I miss a dose? Have a reaction to the medication?
- Are other treatments available?

About Tests . . .

- What kinds of tests are involved?
- What do you expect to find out from these tests?
- When will we know the results?

(continued on next page)

QUESTIONS FOR THE EYE CARE PROFESSIONAL
(*continued*)

- Do I have to do anything special to prepare for any of the tests?
- Do these tests have any side effects or risks?
- Will more tests be necessary later?
- Will you send copies of the results to my doctor?

This list of questions was adapted from the National Eye Institute's tools for talking to an eye care professional, which you can find on the NEI Web site at www.nei.nih.gov/health/talktodoc.asp.

Understanding the physician's responses to your questions is essential. Here are some additional tips for you and your relative:

- Write down your questions ahead of time. If you don't understand your physician's responses, ask questions until you do understand.
- Consider bringing along a friend or family member for support and to help recall the conversation.
- Take notes, or bring a tape recorder to assist in your recollection of the discussion.
- Ask the doctor to write down his or her instructions.
- Ask the doctor for printed material about the condition. If you still have trouble understanding the doctor's answers, ask where you can go for more information.
- Other members of your older relative's health care team, such as nurses and pharmacists, can be good sources of information. Both of you will want to talk to them, too.

If you discover that your relative does have a degree of vision loss, be sure to ask the eye care professional about the appropriateness of low vision services. If he or she cannot refer you to a low vision specialist, consult the sources of information listed in "Getting Help: Where to Start" in Chapter 1.

UNDERSTANDING VISION LOSS FIRSTHAND

People with normal sight can have a difficult time understanding a visually impaired person's description of what he or she can and cannot see. This is a very hard thing to imagine when you have not experienced it yourself, and it is very hard for the person experiencing it to describe. To further complicate matters, many people with vision loss see differently at varied times of the day, or even from day to day. However, trying to imagine what your older relative is experiencing will not only help you assist him or her, it will also probably improve communication and smooth out the potential for conflict. You might want to try out the vision simulators described in the following section to gain insight into your older relatives' experience.

SIMULATING VISION LOSS

Vision simulators are goggles or glasses made of cardboard designed to simulate various visual conditions and show what the individual with a particular eye condition can see. They are often used for training purposes and are available through a number of sources, indicated in the Resources section. However, you might want to make your own simulators for macular degeneration, glaucoma, diabetic retinopathy, or cataracts using the following instructions and using the patterns at the end of this chapter.[3]

INSTRUCTIONS FOR CARDBOARD VISION SIMULATORS

- Photocopy the patterns shown on the following pages.
- Trace the patterns onto poster board.
- Cut out each pattern along the solid lines, including the lines for the eye openings.
- Cut each tab along the solid line down to the dotted line.
- Fold down the tabs, overlapping them slightly and tape them in place with transparent tape. (Overlapping will hold the simulator off the face a little.)
- Pierce holes where indicated and tie strings to the sides of the simulator.

For macular degeneration:
- Cut two pieces of clear plastic about an inch larger than the eye opening, and glue them to the back.
- Cut a circle of dark poster board about an inch smaller than the eye opening.
- Tape the circle to the center of the eye opening so that the person's central vision is blocked off and only a rim of clear plastic remains to see through.

For glaucoma:
- Cut a piece of clear plastic about an inch larger than the small eye opening and glue it to the back.
- When the simulator is worn, the tunnel vision caused by glaucoma will be simulated.

For diabetic retinopathy:
- Cut two pieces of bubble plastic about an inch larger than the eye openings and tape them to the back.
- Color between the bubbles with black and red indelible markers to give the plastic a spotty appearance.
- When the simulator is worn, the spotty, blurred vision caused by diabetic retinopathy will be simulated.

For cataracts:
- Crumple and smooth out a small sheet of wax paper.
- Cut two pieces of wax paper about an inch larger than the eye openings, and glue those to the back.

Try wearing these simulators while doing a variety of tasks such as eating, reading, or walking around the room. They can also be used when checking your older relative's home for hazards (see Chapter 7). Vision rehabilitation professionals—vision rehabilitation therapists and orientation and mobility specialists—use these simulators in their training so they will have a good understanding of what and how people with whom they work may see.

OTHER SOURCES OF SIMULATORS

The following Web sites also show simulations of vision conditions; the last two also have vision simulators available for purchase:

- National Eye Institute (www.nei.nih.gov/photo/index.asp)
- ACBVI Vision Simulation Presentation (www.acbvi.org)
- VisionSimulator.com (www.visionsimulator.com)
- Lighthouse International (www.lighthouse.org/about/low_vision_defined_page2.htm
- Fork in the Road Vision Rehabilitation Services (www.lowvisionsimulators.com)

Recognizing the signs of eye conditions and having a basic understanding of what your older relative is experiencing will help you as you begin to deal with the emotional reactions and adjustments to vision loss. In the next chapter you'll find tips for recognizing and dealing with the many feelings that you and your older relative may experience during the adjustment process.

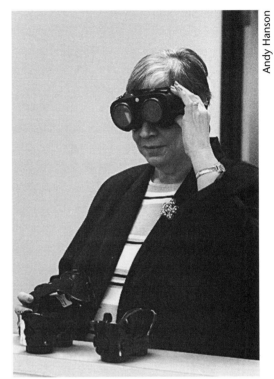

Andy Hanson

Vision simulator goggles or homemade simulators allow you to experience what people with various eye conditions can see.

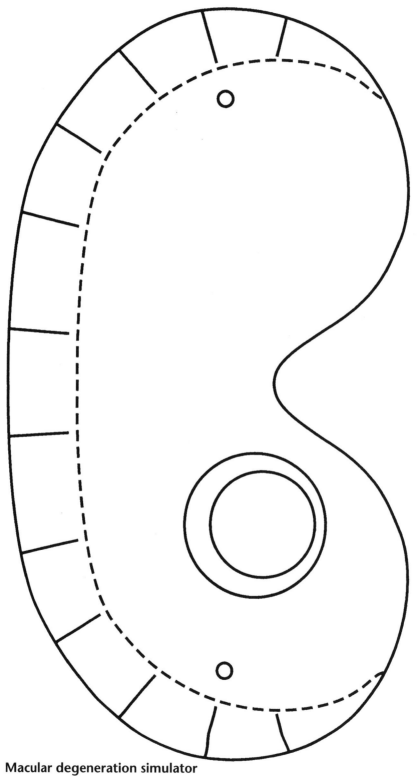

Macular degeneration simulator

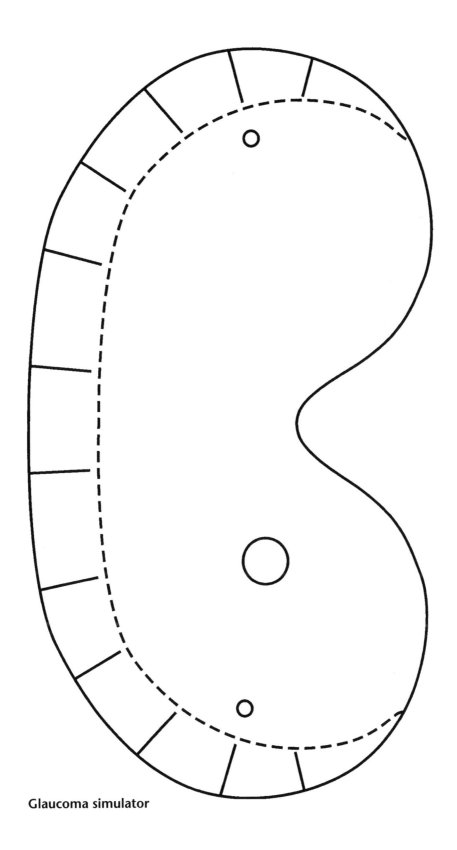

Glaucoma simulator

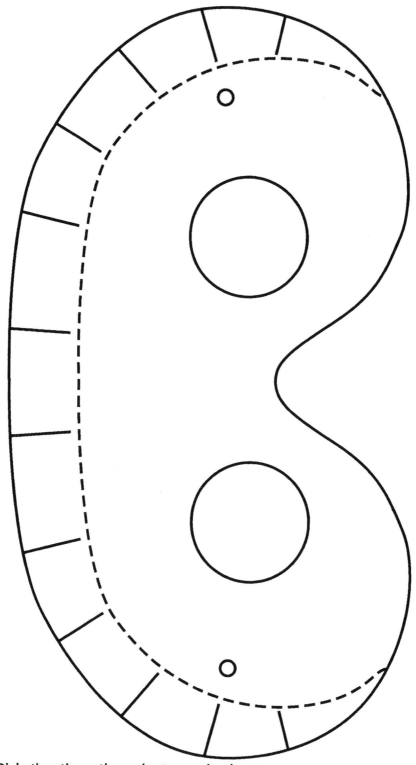

Diabetic retinopathy and cataract simulator

Chapter 3

Emotional Reactions to Vision Loss

After Sandra and her sister figured out that their father, Robert, needed to see an eye care professional, they thought they were out of the woods. Since Robert's wife had passed away three years earlier, Sandra accompanied him to the ophthalmologist's office.

"Finally, Dad's going to get some help," thought Sandra. "We'll have this sorted out in no time."

The ophthalmologist diagnosed Robert's vision problem as macular degeneration. It left a blind spot in the central portion of his vision. Having a name for what Robert was experiencing eased everyone's mind at first. But in the weeks that followed, the reality of the situation set in.

Robert's loss of vision was sudden and severe, and he was left feeling scared, helpless, and frustrated. His daughter felt much the same way, although sometimes her frustration turned into anger. She got mad at her father because he refused to go out of the house except to the doctor. Although Sandra had a busy career, she visited daily and made sure that he had a hot meal and took his medications. Neither of her sisters lived nearby. Every day when she arrived, her father sat in his armchair in his pajamas and robe, refusing to move.

"My life is over," muttered Robert, every time Sandra suggested that he try to become a little more active. "I can't *drive anymore, I can't golf. I can't even cook a decent meal without my eyes. I'm useless."*

Robert didn't seem to be feeling any better as time went on, especially since his ophthalmologist told him that his vision couldn't be improved. As if this weren't enough, his hearing gradually became worse, and he would not consider a hearing aid. Sandra had trouble discussing even routine matters with him. More than once she stormed out of the house at her wits' end.

"Sometimes I get so angry at him," she tearfully told her sister, "and then I get mad at the ophthalmologist for giving us bad news. The other day, I even lost my temper with a cashier in the grocery store—over nothing! Why is this happening to Dad? Why is this happening to us?"

A visit to the doctor and a definitive diagnosis can signal the beginning of your family's adjustment to vision loss, not the end. Vision loss brings with it a whole host of emotional and psychological reactions, and not just to the person experiencing it. The whole family can be affected. All sorts of feelings will crop up for everyone involved, and emotional turmoil at this time is to be expected. You and your loved ones can't avoid these sometimes very difficult feelings—they are natural—and understanding them can help you deal with the situation more effectively. This chapter is intended to help you navigate this emotional terrain, giving you some insight into your older relative's experiences and helping you sort out your own complex reactions. Adjusting to change isn't easy, but can be done.

THE CHALLENGES OF AGING

As we all grow older, we face a number of challenging adjustments and losses. Some of the typical losses that people face as they age include the following:
- Loss of a spouse or significant other
- Loss of siblings, neighbors, close friends, and peers
- Loss of geographic proximity to children, grandchildren, and longtime friends

- Loss of peak physical or cognitive functioning
- Loss of good health due to chronic disease or acute illness
- Loss of work and its accompanying satisfactions
- Loss of financial security

Your awareness of experiences and concerns that may be troubling your older relative can help you understand his or her behavior and emotional reactions in the face of vision loss.

As people grow older, they often experience very painful changes, such as the end of a career or death of a spouse, siblings, or close friends. People whom they count on and care about, and who, perhaps equally important, understand them, are suddenly gone, and they can feel as if they are lost and alone. These changes can have a profound impact and fuel the feeling that things probably will never return to normal. Some individuals begin to realize that they have to invent a whole new idea of normal—to transform their lives and expectations.

On top of losing very significant individuals in their lives, many older people often do not have the comfort of having children, grandchildren, and other family and friends close by. In today's mobile society, moving away for jobs, school, and many other reasons is common.

Changes in health and financial status are also frequent experiences. Health is something we usually take for granted until we begin to experience problems. As we grow older, we may find ourselves dealing with the discomfort and sometimes the indignities of even minor problems, much less life-threatening illnesses, that can be coupled with other obstacles. For example, physical problems such as hearing loss can make it difficult to communicate, while memory loss can make coping with other losses and learning new skills challenging.

Loss of financial security is something that can result from the loss of a spouse, or from retirement, illness, a turn in the stock market, or spending down one's retirement savings. And losing one's vision or hearing can be an additional expense. Medicare, for example, does not pay for adaptive equipment and devices associated with vision or hearing problems.

All these changes are difficult, but the feeling of loss of control that many older persons experience may be the hardest challenge they face. Being unable to drive a car, for example, after having been mobile all one's life, can be a serious blow. Having been independent for so long, an older person can become angry or depressed when faced with these new realities of life. It is against this backdrop that many older people experience vision loss, which can exacerbate and intensify all these feelings.

COMMON REACTIONS TO VISUAL LOSS

The challenges brought about by loss of vision can seem overwhelming to both the older person and his or her family. Many strong feelings can develop at this time, including fear, shock, anger, and depression.[1] Before people have a chance to adjust and receive professional support and until they learn adaptive techniques to help them continue their daily activities, they may feel a variety of negative emotions.

Some people who experience vision loss may initially lose their sense of self-worth and self-confidence because—at least at first—they may not be able to engage in daily activities without assistance. The roles and responsibilities that they have traditionally assumed come under threat; volunteer and recreational activities might be affected as well. Even normal household tasks can become difficult for some people, and shame, embarrassment, and feelings of inadequacy may result. Your mother, for example, might feel uncomfortable because she can no longer read her mail and pay her bills without someone helping with these personal matters. Or she may feel unable to clean her house adequately because she can't see whether she is doing a good job.

Sometimes, older persons who experience vision loss can lose some of their friends, because being around someone with a disability makes some people uncomfortable. Some may even feel that vision loss is contagious. Friends frequently do not know what to do or say to a person who can no longer see well and end up avoiding the situation altogether. On the other hand, sometimes older people with vision loss feel embarrassed and want to avoid friends and acquaintances. They may feel uncomfortable going out in public for meals or leisure activities and may turn down invitations so many times that friends stop asking. The

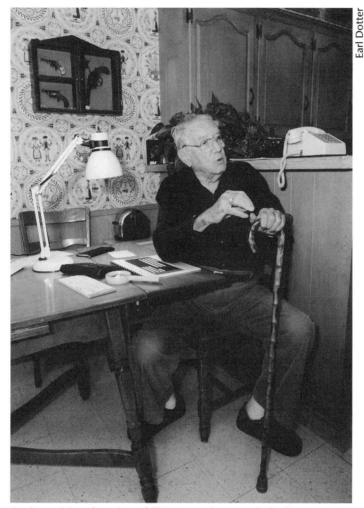

Earl Dotter

Facing vision loss in addition to the usual challenges of aging can lead many older people to feel fearful and depressed. But beginning to learn the special skills that can help them take care of everyday tasks, such as paying bills, can begin to restore their self-confidence and self-esteem.

resulting isolation can lead to feelings of loneliness and even depression.

The stigma of vision loss can weigh heavily on those experiencing it as well. Because of the prevalence of negative stereotypes in our culture, people fear being labeled as "that blind person." For example, they may refuse to use the long white cane that helps many visually impaired people get around safely because it might identify them as being "blind" and, perhaps, "not normal."

"My mother became very depressed and even suicidal as a result of her loss of vision from glaucoma. The rehabilitation center helped her tremendously by teaching her how to adjust to being blind and by keeping her so busy that she had no time to focus on her blindness."

—Page R., Atlanta

Mistaken notions about blindness and vision loss can restrict them all the more and initiate a vicious circle: being limited by a condition, having negative feelings about it, and limiting oneself even more than is necessary. Becoming depressed about a disability can become an additional disability in and of itself.

In addition, some of the challenges that accompany a physical condition can magnify those that come from vision loss. In the case of Robert Mackinnon, for instance, having a hearing impairment worsened the effects of vision loss. However, it can help you and your family members to be aware that just as physical rehabilitation services can help individuals who have had a stroke, older individuals with vision loss may be helped through vision rehabilitation professionals and services. Many of the challenges of vision loss can be met successfully through consultation with trained rehabilitation professionals. You might feel as if you need to handle everything yourself, but there are a lot of resources that you and your family can draw on. (See Chapter 1, and for detailed information about the kind of services that are available, see Chapter 5.)

YOUR RELATIVE'S EMOTIONAL RESPONSES TO VISION LOSS

Reactions to vision loss can be profound, and some experts have likened them to the stages of grieving after the death of a loved one that have been described by Elizabeth Kübler-Ross.[2] These responses, which might not be experienced in this particular order, include

- denial
- depression
- anger

- bargaining
- acceptance

You and members of your family may also go through your own grieving process and experience an array of feelings in reaction to your relative's vision loss. You may feel angry, helpless, frustrated, guilty, and unable to cope as well.

Just like Robert Mackinnon, your relative may have a variety of feelings, including wanting to just give up. One common reaction to vision loss is fear—of the unknown, of the inability to continue to do daily tasks, of loss of independence, and of helplessness. Another reaction is anger—perhaps toward God or fate for inflicting this loss, or toward doctors, or friends and family members. Anger can often be directed toward those we love the most and can even be turned inward and result in depression.

Grief and mourning are frequent responses, as is denial that a vision problem even exists at all. Sometimes people act out their denial by going from doctor to doctor to search of a more positive diagnosis; others may isolate themselves physically or mentally and can become depressed. Other reactions can include embarrassment or self-consciousness about perceived limited abilities, despair, devastation, exhaustion from emotional turmoil, and even surprise that such a situation could occur.

Given everyone's possible emotional turmoil, misunderstandings may arise and communication may become especially complicated when family members have a difficult time being open and honest about the changes in family dynamics caused by the onset of vision loss. You and your family may feel uncertain about when to talk directly about the loss with your older relative, but communication can be key in helping everyone begin to connect with each other, solve problems, and adjust. (See the chapter that follows for tips on how to communicate effectively.) In addition, there are a variety of strategies that can help your older relative at this difficult time (see "Facing Vision Loss: Helping Your Relative Begin to Adjust").

The majority of people may become depressed as they adjust to vision loss, but some can remain depressed for a prolonged period. It is important that family members be aware of changes in their

FACING VISION LOSS: HELPING YOUR RELATIVE BEGIN TO ADJUST

When someone experiences vision loss, emotional turmoil can be felt by everyone in the family. In addition to trying to deal with any number of powerful emotions, family members may be affected by changes that will need to take place. Chapters 1 and 5 offer suggestions on how to find immediate help, Chapters 6 and 7 provide numerous practical tips on how someone's home and activities can be adjusted to maintain an independent life, and other strategies outlined in this chapter can be helpful in moving the person with vision loss and the entire family out of initial shock and fear and into a manageable new reality. The following suggestions may begin to help you and your older relative on your way to adjustment.

1. Help your older relative build self-confidence by helping him or her succeed at a task he or she has always done well. For example, if your mother has always been complimented on making the best chocolate cake in the neighborhood, she can still do that—with some encouragement and a few helpful tips on how to adapt her kitchen and her techniques. (See Chapters 6 and 7 and the Resources section in the back of this book.)

2. Support your relative's self-esteem and confidence by encouraging him or her to try doing things in a new and different way. For example, your father may have always loved to read novels and may be despondent that he cannot see well enough to read anymore. Encourage him to try Talking Books. Be sure to mention how much your friends are enjoying listening to books in their cars or as they go out walking or jogging because they are too busy to sit down and read a print book.

3. Stay focused on helping your relative find solutions to everyday problems as needed. Instead of letting yourself be overwhelmed by how your uncle is going to continue to live all alone since he has experienced vision loss, start by helping him accomplish one task at a time, such as shaving or making coffee, and learning how to adapt as he goes.

4. Try to be supportive without being patronizing. If your mother is going to try baking her famous cake, offer help and encouragement but don't attempt to take over for her. Offer assistance if she wants it, but don't

---

FACING VISION LOSS (*continued*)

start doing everything for her. Also, try to be sensitive to the tone of voice you use. She may perceive that you are just humoring her and you really think she can't do it.

5. Keep the lines of communication open. If your father stops calling you or is abrupt with you after you suggest hiring a housekeeper—when he was the one who complained about not being able to see to clean the house properly—try to reopen the conversation, talk about his feelings, and suggest other possible alternatives. (Also see Chapter 4 on family communication.)

6. Address issues on a regular basis so your relative knows you are continually concerned and so that they can be dealt with one at a time. For example, if you notice that the food in the refrigerator that you purchased or prepared has not been eaten, find out why. Your aunt might not be able to locate the food in the refrigerator, might be uneasy cooking it on the stove or in the microwave, or might be depressed and not feel like eating. Each of these possibilities can be dealt with—but each calls for a different solution.

7. Ask for help from your relative when you need it. For example, your father may be a champ at doing tax returns, and you may be hopelessly lost. He would probably be delighted to help you—if you explain the forms and any changes that the Internal Revenue Service may have made.

8. Remember to take care of yourself by continuing to pay attention to yourself and your own life! You'll feel better and will be better able to help your relative too.

To find out more about what resources and services are available to help you and your older relative deal with issues related to vision loss, see Chapter 5 and the Resources section of this book.

---

older relative's emotional state and also watch out for depression in themselves. Some signs that might signal depression are:
- changes in sleeping patterns, weight, or behavior
- lack of appetite
- excessive worry
- lack of interest in activities, events, or people
- bouts of crying

- lack of motivation, or apathy, listlessness, or general disinterest
- overall pessimism and moping
- refusal to communicate or social withdrawal[3]

Prolonged depression should not be ignored. If you observe signs of depression in your older relative, do not hesitate to talk to him or her about it. Make sure he or she knows that you are aware of his or her feelings and that you want to help. In many instances, professional help may be important, with counseling and possibly the prescription of antidepressant medication. If your family has a religious affiliation, it can be helpful to re-member that a member of the clergy might also be a source of support. The important point is to pay attention to the emotions you and your family members are experiencing and seek help if necessary.

If your older relative has not yet gotten involved in a vision rehabilitation program, this might be a good time to suggest that he or she get started. (Chapter 5 deals specifically with how to lo-cate professional help and rehabilitation services.) If depression is preventing your older relative from taking action, professional assistance may be all the more critical. It may be easier at first to make an appointment for your older relative with a primary care physician, who if necessary can make a referral to a trained men-tal health clinician. If you do so, you might want to alert the doctor from the outset to the possibility of depression.

It is important however, to recognize that some older people will not be receptive to this type of clinical intervention, in which case encouraging them to become involved in vision re-habilitation may be most helpful. If a vision rehabilitation pro-fessional can help your older relative realize that he or she can still continue to do just one valued activity, such as pouring a liquid without spilling by using a special device or reading with a magnifier, it can encourage him or her to continue with a reha-bilitation program, which can often alleviate depression.

YOUR EMOTIONS

While trying to attend to your older relative's needs, you may ex-perience any of a number of feelings and reactions of your own. In the scenario at the beginning of this chapter, Sandra was frustrated and felt she could do very little for her father because he did not want to do anything for himself. Maybe she even found it difficult to imagine her father as needing help and was angry at him for not appearing strong or in control—qualities she believed a father should still have. Although complicated and hard to cope with, Sandra's feelings and experiences are normal and natural.

You may have your own feelings about your older relative wanting or needing to rely on you heavily. You might be overwhelmed with pressures to get everything done, and feel guilty when you can't manage everything at once. At times, you may be experiencing conflicting feelings. Although you may genuinely want to be helpful and supportive, you might feel resentful of the time involved. Your personality, values, coping strategies, and family dynamic will influence how you feel. But keep in mind that your feelings are not out of the ordinary, and remembering that may help prevent you from becoming overwhelmed by what you feel. Your own mental health is as important as your relative's. Seek counseling or other support if you need it. Being aware of these and a number of other points can be helpful in getting through tough moments and a difficult period of time (see "Facing Vision Loss: Helping Yourself"). One of them is realizing that most people experience similar reactions when someone in their family becomes visually impaired.

DENIAL OF VISION LOSS

"I became really depressed when I found out about my mother's vision loss. At first I denied it." Just as the older person with vision loss may have difficulty accepting what has happened, family members may experience denial as well. They may choose not to believe that their mother or father has permanently lost some sight and may persist in visiting doctor after doctor for new diagnoses or treatments. They may want to ignore the realities of vision loss and treat the older person as a sighted

> **"I became really depressed when I found out about my mother's vision loss. At first I denied it; then I shed some tears and wondered what could be done."**
> —*Robbin T., Atlanta*

FACING VISION LOSS: HELPING YOURSELF

Vision loss, whether experienced by a relative or friend or oneself, can seem overwhelming. If you feel this way, you're not alone. Reacting to vision loss with a range of strong, often negative feelings is understandable, and it is an experience shared at first by just about everyone in similar circumstances. In trying to regain some equilibrium, you may find that keeping in mind the following points may help:

- Allow yourself and your relative time. It is the element that often makes the difference in life. No matter what is happening or how things seem, nothing lasts forever. Learning about vision loss and adjusting to it constitute an ongoing process. You're in transition, and it may be helpful to remember just that.

- Emotional support from people who care about you is critical. Although you may be tired or tend to withdraw when you feel less than perfect, try to stay in touch with friends and other people who can boost your spirits and provide assistance.

- Do your best to pay attention to what matters to *you*, even though you may sometimes feel too tired to do so. You're entitled to take care of your own life without feeling guilty. Taking care of *yourself*—eating what's good for you, sleeping as much as you can, relaxing or doing activities that are important to you—is your first job. It can help you maintain your spirits and strength and in that way help your older relative too.

- When you don't understand your relative's feelings, reactions, or behavior, try to put yourself in his or her place. Trying to see something through another person's perspective can help you deal with the situation at hand and support a better relationship.

- Become informed about your relative's eye condition and about services and help that may be of use to you and your family. Most people are aware that the Internet is a great source of information, and you can find out about a wealth of resources by using it. You may not be aware, though, of the variety of national organizations that offer information, support, and referrals to visually impaired people and their families. In addition, a number of publications offer invaluable advice. (See Chapters 1 and 5 and the Resources section of this book.)

FACING VISION LOSS (*continued*)

- Try to identify and consult with professionals who are knowledgeable about your relative's eye condition, and establish an ongoing relationship with a doctor and other service providers you feel you can trust. Friends, colleagues, and your own health care providers can be sources of information about professionals. University-affiliated hospitals, professional organizations, and national organizations in the field of vision loss can also provide valuable suggestions.
- If you need help dealing with the challenges that you are experiencing, don't hesitate to consult professionals for support and advice. Support groups for family members can be the most helpful resource during difficult times, when it may seem as though the only people who understand what you're going through are people who have been there too (see Chapter 5). Such support groups can be located through national organizations; local hospitals, other health care facilities, and social service agencies; and religious organizations as well.

person. Once people learn about available vision-related services, and have a chance to begin adjusting to this dramatic change in the family, their feelings of denial may begin to dissipate.

FEAR OR SADNESS

You may find that you are frightened about what vision loss will mean to you and your family and be anxious about what the future may hold. You may also find yourself feeling sad or depressed about your older relative's eye condition. Some people may think about "how Mom used to be," and this sadness may even turn into grieving. You might also begin to feel concerned about what the future holds for you in particular, especially if your relative's eye condition is hereditary. When this is the case, consider sharing your thoughts and feelings with people who can understand and be supportive. Discussing fears about your own eyesight with knowledgeable professionals such as eye care professionals or genetic counselors can also help you deal with difficult issues.

ANGER OR CONFUSION

Family members can feel angry or confused about their relative's vision loss and react with annoyance when the person with a visual impairment has his or her own reactions, such as insisting that the furniture or objects like clothing or food not be moved. They may not realize at first that shifting an object just a few inches may result in the older person's falling or having to search for an item that he or she needs.

> "I wake up very angry sometimes about having to take over being the parent. I feel stuck."
>
> –Judy R., Atlanta

Also, some family members may resent that shopping or other everyday chores can take the older person so much longer than before, and they may need time to adjust to these and other new realities.

GUILT AND RESENTMENT

Some people may feel guilty about their own behavior or their perceived failings in the face of vision loss, such as not being able to find the right doctor who can "fix" their older relative's eye problem. They may think they have to take over for their older relative and may feel bad about having busy lives and not spending more time with their mother or father. Relationships can become strained when their parent may, in turn, say or do things that contribute to the guilt that they are feeling. Often, guilt can turn into resentment. When feelings run this high, it may be helpful to talk to supportive friends or airing these feelings may help relieve them.

NOT UNDERSTANDING VISION LOSS

"Neither my brother or I had any idea of the impact of vision loss on our mother. We thought she'd just be able to figure out how to cope, adjust, and go on as she always has." Perhaps you can identify with those thoughts—or these:

"Some of my family, who don't live with my father, don't

know what to do. They sometimes treat him as if he's crazy or not a whole person. They just don't know how to handle being around a person who's visually impaired."

When people haven't encountered someone with a visual impairment or had a reason to learn about vision loss, they may expect their older relative to continue to behave as before. They may not understand that the older person's vision may fluctuate on a daily basis or realize what this fluctuation means to the person's ability to function when he or she fails to react to visual cues or recognize familiar faces, they may not understand what is happening.

Similarly, at first you may not have comprehended why your older relative no longer turned on the television or used the microwave. You may not realize immediately that you cannot leave notes in regular-sized handwriting on the refrigerator door and expect your older relative to be able to read them. As you begin to understand more about your older relative's eye condition, many misunderstandings can be alleviated.

EMBARRASSMENT ABOUT VISION LOSS

An older person's vision loss can cause embarrassment to his or her family, some of whom may want to avoid being seen in public with the person. They may feel uncomfortable if their older relative makes a mistake, such as putting on a blouse and skirt that do not match, or not immediately recognizing someone they know quite well. Activities such as taking the older person to the grocery store or eating out in public may be stressful when people feel embarrassed or self-conscious about their older relative's behavior stemming from diminished vision. Although such feelings may take time to recede, when the older relative begins to learn skills or techniques for performing daily activities, the family in general may begin to feel more relaxed.

MAKING ASSUMPTIONS ABOUT THE OLDER PERSON'S CAPABILITIES

When someone develops vision loss, the family can jump to a number of conclusions. Although some people overestimate the

"I try not to say 'It's too dangerous' to my dad when he is trying to do something."

–Linda B., Boston

capabilities of their visually impaired relative, others underestimate them. You may be concerned about the safety of your father if he chooses to continue to cook for himself or carry out other household chores. You might be worried that he will burn himself or even set the house on fire. To protect him, you might even insist on preparing meals and doing his laundry, and hire a part- or full-time professional caregiver. However, vision rehabilitation professionals can teach him skills to help him function normally and independently, even in the kitchen.

Sometimes family members may assume that their visually impaired mother is not safe at home and may worry about her falling or hurting herself—particularly in the bathroom or on the stairs. They may conclude that she can no longer remain in her own home. With the proper rehabilitation skills training, however, having the older person move to a family member's home or a residential facility is usually not really necessary.

UNCERTAINTY ABOUT HOW MUCH IS ENOUGH

Many family members often feel uncertain about when to help and when to step back. Although you may be concerned about limiting your older relative's independence by helping too much, you might also worry that you aren't doing enough. You might be uncomfortable watching your aunt blunder as she practices her new skills or becomes disoriented. Keep in mind that you need to afford your older relative the time to learn by making some mistakes.

An older person's feelings of uncertainty and the family's concerns about him or her can lead some family members to assume the role of parent to their own parent. Although some changes in family roles may be unavoidable, thinking that the roles of parent and child can be reversed is probably not helpful for anyone involved. Try to address these feelings directly in family discussions, but if doing so seems beyond you, the aid of a trained counselor can be of great benefit.

HANDLING YOUR REACTIONS

You, your siblings, and other family members may experience these or other reactions to the visual impairment of your older relative. Try to remember that they are all normal and that services are available to help you, your family, and your older relative adjust. Professionals will also be able to offer you concrete suggestions for enabling your older relative to remain as independent as possible. (See Chapters 6 and 7 for some specific suggestions.) You may also find that during this transitional time, as you, your relative, and other members of your family begin to adjust to this new set of life circumstances, adjusting your behavior to accommodate your relative's vision loss is helpful and important (see "Facing Vision Loss: Tips for Family and Friends"). Finally, if you feel that you are experiencing negative or intense reactions over a prolonged period of time, do not hesitate to get some assistance from a trained clinical professional, which may be helpful as well for your older relative. The sooner you are feeling supported, the sooner you may be able to think more constructively about how best to assist your relative. This can create the best-case scenario for everyone.

FACING VISION LOSS: TIPS FOR FAMILY AND FRIENDS

When a member of the family experiences vision loss, everyone can benefit from remembering that certain adjustments in behavior and expectations are important. When someone can no longer see as well as before, personal interactions and daily activities may need to take this new reality into account. The following are simple pointers that can help everyone and can be shared with friends as well as family:

- **Identify yourself to the older person with vision loss.** Say hello first to your older relative and identify yourself. Especially when initially adjusting to vision loss, he or she may not recognize everyone's voice in every situation. You can avoid awkwardness for everyone by simply saying,

(continued on next page)

FACING VISION LOSS (*continued*)

"Hi, Uncle Robert, it's Joan." If the person no longer needs you to introduce yourself, you can stop doing so.

- **Don't walk away without telling the person that you are leaving the immediate environment.** If your relative can't see you, he or she may not realize you are gone. He or she may even continue to talk to you, as though you're still present, and this can cause embarrassment and a number of other feelings.

- **Talk directly to the person.** Sometimes people unconsciously begin speaking differently to people with impairments, particularly in social situations. It's as though the person isn't really there at all. Don't ask Uncle Robert's daughter how Uncle Robert is feeling today or what he would like to drink. Ask him directly. It's surprising how "invisible" people with vision or hearing loss can become, simply because those around them may feel uncomfortable.

- **It's okay to use words like "see" or "look."** These words are part of normal vocabulary, and there's no need to be afraid of using them. Everyday conversation does not need to change. For example, it's perfectly fine to say, "Did you see your friend George yesterday?"

- **Give clear and specific directions, taking vision loss into consideration.** Don't provide information that is based on someone's ability to see, such as, "Your coat is over there." Be more specific, for example, "Your coat is on a chair just to the left of the desk, about 2 feet in front of you."

- **Communicate verbally and avoid relying on nonverbal expressions.** Similarly, your older relative may not be able to see you make certain gestures, such as shrugging your shoulders or using a "thumbs up" sign to communicate. He or she also might not be able to see the smile on your face that indicates you are teasing when you make certain comments.

- **Don't move anything around without asking.** The simple movement of a chair or coffee table may cause a problem for your relative. He may be using the chair as a landmark for getting around, or she may bump into the coffee table if it is moved. If small objects, such as medications or house keys are moved from their designated places, he or she may not be able to find them again.

FACING VISION LOSS (*continued*)

- **Make your writing readable.** Your relative might not be able to see a note you have left if you write with a regular pen and in normal handwriting. Get in the habit of using black felt-tip markers and printing clearly. Some people with vision loss can read large print if it is printed in large, dark letters or typed in 18-point or larger type. Ask what works for your relative. (For "Tips for Print Readability," see Chapter 10.)

- **If you notice a spot on your relative's clothing, or something else about his or her appearance, take him or her aside and let him or her know.** People generally appreciate it if someone tactfully and discretely lets them know about something wrong with their appearance, and in all likelihood your relative would want to know about this as much as anyone else. Similarly, there might be times when you need to explain privately that your relative's clothes don't match. (You might want to offer to help label matching items in the closet or dresser to avoid this type of situation in the future, as explained in Chapter 7.)

- **Learn how to walk safely with a person who is visually impaired.** A simple technique called sighted guide described in Chapter 6 is used when someone who is visually impaired needs to be guided by someone else who can see. The technique allows everyone to feel more relaxed and reassured, and once the older person learns this technique he or she can teach friends how to walk comfortably with him or her.

- **Learn about products that can help your relative continue to do everyday tasks and enjoyable activities independently.** Talking or large-print watches, clocks, thermometers, calculators, and scales are just a few of the products that have been adapted for people with vision loss. Using them can make a tremendous amount of difference. These adaptive devices make great birthday or holiday gift ideas for friends and relatives, as do large-print playing cards, games, calendars, and address books. You can also consider giving your relative a book on tape or disk, or, if you are a close family member, assist in the purchase of a reading device such as a closed-circuit television system (CCTV). (See Chapters 6 and 7 and the Resources section.)

- **In general, ask first before helping, and allow your relative to do as much as he or she can independently.** Treat your older relative with dignity, just as you would like to be treated.

ADJUSTMENT

Adjustment to vision loss is an individual matter. The pace at which your older relative adjusts depends on many factors, such as his or her ability to cope with challenging situations and the involvement, reactions, and support of family members and close friends. The adjustment process varies and for some it may be a slow process.

The older person's health can be a factor as well. Your relative's perceptions and attitudes about aging, disabilities, and vision loss also enter into the adjustment process. For example, some older persons who lose vision later in life have accepted stereotypes about aging and vision loss. They may believe that persons who are visually impaired must be taken care of, or that "you can't teach an old dog new tricks." Beliefs such as these are myths that need to be overcome as part of adjusting.

For older people, making the psychological adjustment to vision loss may be more difficult than the ability to accept other losses.[4] Learning new ways of doing things can be interesting and challenging, but actually accepting that vision loss is permanent can be very difficult for some people. The onset of vision loss can bring to the surface negative attitudes ingrained by one's culture, or society, which can make adjustment even harder.[5] But taking steps like finding out about essential vision rehabilitation services and working with professional counselors can move everyone toward more positive attitudes. It is not uncommon for the whole family to go through this process—either together or individually.

Chapter 4

Family Dynamics: On the Road to Adjustment

The last time Emil Vasquez visited his mother, Delores, he ended up leaving her apartment in a huff. Although he visited her to see if he could help her with some chores around the house, his mother got angry and shooed him out a half hour after he arrived. Ever since Delores had been diagnosed with glaucoma, Emil had felt helpless. He was upset that his mother would not let him help out, and he was puzzled why she always seemed to get angry with him. It wasn't like her.

Today, Emil stopped by his mother's apartment just to talk. He wanted to understand better what was happening and let his mother know what he was feeling.

"I wanted to talk with you a little bit about last week, if that's okay," Emil began a little stiffly. "I was trying to be helpful, cleaning up some papers and photos in that big pile in the living room, and then all of a sudden you got mad and made me leave. I just couldn't understand why. I was worried you would trip over that stuff on the floor and hurt yourself. I even took the afternoon off work to do it. I'm sorry if I upset you. I didn't mean to."

"Well, son, I appreciate you wanting to help," Delores said slowly. "It's just that last week you didn't even call me before you showed up. I would have tried to clean up a little first if I had known you were coming over. And then you just started moving things around without asking. Because of my glaucoma,

I couldn't even see what you were doing at first. Those things you were 'cleaning up' were some important papers I was going over, plus a lot of family pictures. When I realized you were putting them somewhere and I might not be able to find them again, I got so upset. I asked you to stop, but I thought that you weren't even answering me. I realized later that I didn't have my hearing aid in. I guess I started yelling because I didn't think you could hear me."

Emil and Delores both looked as if a weight had been lifted from their shoulders. They sat back and continued to talk about how they might avoid misunderstandings like this in the future. Then they began to sort through the family photos together.

By now you may be thinking that the onset of vision loss can often make everyone in your family feel as though the world is being turned upside down. In addition to the strong and possibly disturbing feelings various family members may have, many changes and disruptions may be taking place, and numerous unknowns seem to be intruding on life as you thought you knew it. During times of turmoil, it may not be easy for people to step back, breathe deeply, and think about the best way in which to deal with a complex challenge, but that may be just what is most helpful.

When anyone experiences powerful emotions and confusion runs high, it often becomes difficult to think clearly and make effective decisions. But trying to understand what you are feeling and what you want to accomplish—as well as what your older relative may be feeling and what he or she wants to accomplish—can be a good place to begin to deal with the situation. At this point, good communication can make all the difference.

COMMUNICATION: THE HEART OF THE MATTER

Effective communication, where all parties understand each other, can help people see eye to eye. That is, agreements can be reached, and in those cases in which they cannot, each person nevertheless is clear about the thoughts and desires of the other. That clarity can set the stage for more useful discussions and agreement down the road. Powerful emotions can act as a roadblock to productive communication, yet we typically need each other's support the most when we are feeling emotionally vulnerable. Ironically, it is just those times when clear communication is threatened that it is also the most critical. As your family comes to terms with vision loss, it will be helpful to remember that communicating with your older relative with sensitivity and empathy is of great importance. You might not always find it easy to be sen-

"Vision loss is difficult to experience and many people fear it. There are periods of adjustment when family members may not understand or appreciate what a vision loss is like to deal with. Time will bring adjustment, as will learning new skills together. Communication between family members is the answer."

–Joseph and Anna Mary R.,
Pennsylvania

sitive or empathetic, especially when stress and negative feelings may have gotten the better of you. However, few things will help you more than taking your relative's perspective into account and trying to imagine what he or she is experiencing. Pay attention to your own emotions as well. Stepping back and understanding your own feelings can prevent you from saying something out of anger or frustration. Overall, knowing yourself will make you a better communicator. Keeping a number of other principles in mind will be valuable as well.

TIPS FOR EFFECTIVE COMMUNICATION

Talking to your older relative about personal issues may be difficult, since you both may be accustomed to a relationship where you are the one going to him or her for help, rather than the other way around. But just because he or she may be in a vulnerable situation, it does not mean that he or she now needs to be treated like a child by you, the adult. Your relative still draws on a wealth of life experiences as a mature human being.

Sometimes, situations may arise where you will be at odds with other family members as well. For instance, suppose your brother, who lives a good distance away, pays your mother a visit. He might offer her a great deal of advice without knowing about or really understanding the complex issues that you and your mother have been discussing. In circumstances like these, effective communication can benefit everyone.

The following suggestions may help you and your family members talk effectively with each other:

- **Keep the lines of communication open.** You may want to say something to your older relative but hesitate instead. Holding back can create tension and emotional undercurrents that make everyone uncomfortable. But what we don't say can frequently get in the way with what we do want to say. Think through what and how you want to communicate, and then say it clearly and with as much sensitivity as you can.

- **Try to overcome your fear of discussing difficult information.** Because you may be worried about upsetting your older relative, from time to time you may find yourself thinking, "How in the world can I broach *this* topic?" Keep in mind, though, that many people are not as fragile or touchy as we perceive them to be. Your relative might even surprise you by speaking openly in response, glad to know what the problem really is. Suppose, for example, you want to say something like this to your mother, "You know, the doctor said you have macular degeneration, which came as a shock to both of us. Sometimes when I get news like that, I can't remember anything anyone says afterward. Were you able to hear what Dr. Jackson said about what you can expect to be able to see?" Although you may be afraid of your mother's reaction to such a direct statement about her condition, she might surprise you by replying, "Well, I'm not happy, but I know other people with macular degeneration, and they've learned to live with it. They got help, and I will too."

- **When you have something difficult to say, prepare ahead of time.** Think about how you feel and what you want the outcome of the conversation to be. Knowing your feelings and goals and organizing your thoughts can have a profound effect on the discussions you have with your relative about vision loss. Conversations handled thoughtfully can make big differences, for example, getting someone to agree to visit a doctor rather than avoiding the issue.

- **Break the ice.** Bring up ideas incrementally and when the moment seems most appropriate. Don't overwhelm your relative with too many different issues at once. You might say, for example, "You know, I've been thinking about all the services and devices that the doctor said were available, but we probably ought to start with one thing at a time. Why don't we begin with the low vision specialist? It sounds like he would be able to show you some things that would help you with what you want to do everyday. Do you think that might help you feel a little better?"

- **Be straightforward and direct.** Speaking directly will help your relative feel that he or she can be honest and open with you too. Directly confronting tough topics that need to be discussed can be the best way to get through difficult times, even though it may be somewhat uncomfortable, especially at first. You could begin by saying, for example, "I want to tell you how important it is for you to make that appointment for that low vision evaluation the ophthalmologist recommended. I'm guessing you may be feeling discouraged, but don't give up yet. It sounds like this appointment might really help you, and I think we should take advantage of it."

- **But be sensitive too!** You can be direct while still being sensitive. Try to be aware of your relative's circumstances and how he or she might be feeling. Your tone of voice matters: *How* you say something is as important as what you say. Sometimes, our tone, manner, body language, and behavior can communicate even more than our words.

- **When communicating, give your relative your full attention.** Talking meaningfully with someone is difficult when we're in the middle of doing something else. Not only can we miss a lot of important information, but the person we're talking with can sometimes feel as if we really don't care what he or she is saying. Speak directly to your relative, and stay focused on the conversation. Don't try, for instance, to converse while you're looking through the mail or checking what's cooking on the stove.

- **Communicate your feelings about a situation.** Letting your relative know—tactfully—what you're feeling can be helpful during the adjustment process. Not only can it relieve tension you might be feeling, but it might also help your older relative understand you better. A calm and sympathetic tone helps too, such as, "You know I'm happy to spend time with you and help out with things around the house, but the kids need me too. So does Angela. We're just going to try to figure out a situation that's good for all of us, okay?"

- **Postpone difficult conversations when emotions are running too high.** It's hard to accomplish anything when we are upset. Sometimes you may need to wait to have important discussions until you and your relative are calmer. When tempers flare, things can be said that everyone regrets later. It's probably best to cool off before discussing tough issues, such as whether it might be best for your relative to move in with you. If you're both crying, focus on your grief at that moment instead of tackling the logistics of how to start a vision rehabilitation program. Communicate your feelings; try not to let them shut down your communications.

- **Be supportive.** Whatever specific challenges your relative might be facing in adjusting to vision loss, the most important message you'll want to convey is that you want to support him or her. For example, when you offer to take your mother to a low vision appointment, don't end the offer with a comment like, "But I just don't know how I'm going to find the time." Instead, try to be direct and supportive: "Mom, this is a busy time for me. I'll gladly make the appointment, but we may have to wait a couple of weeks until the kids go back to school. Maybe your friend Mrs. Gilley could take you if you want to go right away. I really would like to go with you myself, though, so I can learn more about low vision. I want to help you as much as I can. What do you think?"

- **Ask your relative for help when you need to.** You may need help as well, so don't be afraid to ask. In fact, being able to help you in return might make it easier for your relative to accept your assistance. Maybe your father could babysit for you while you run an errand for him. Or you might say to your mother, "George loves your amazing biscuits. Could you make some dough for me to take home?"

- **Promote mutual understanding.** Sometimes, two people walk away from a discussion with completely different ideas about what was communicated. Before ending a conversation, it's useful to check to make sure that both of you understood what was said. One way to do that is to recap the conversation—or see if your relative can: "So, what do you think about what I said about the low vision specialist? Do you think it's a good place to start?"

SOMETIMES, NO EASY ANSWERS

Although communication can be the key to working out and through difficult situations, it's also true that communication alone can't solve every problem. But it can help! When you and your relative don't seem to be able to work out decisions or courses of action easily, try not to be discouraged but to give it some time. Sometimes people need time to deal with their feelings and fears and get used to new challenges; sometimes they need to gather information and absorb it; sometimes they need to speak with friends and acquaintances and think about what they want to do.

When trying to discuss tough issues or deal with frightening

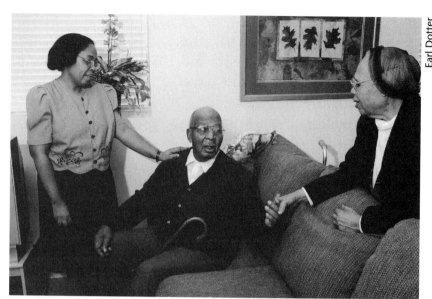

Earl Dotter

As your family comes to terms with vision loss, communicating clearly and directly, but with sensitivity and empathy, is of great importance.

or intimidating circumstances, it's also useful to remember that when we communicate with people, we usually have a few basic needs or goals that we'd like to be met. Typically, we want the other person to understand what we're saying and to assimilate whatever information we're trying to offer. For instance, if you think your father may be developing glaucoma, you may want him to understand what glaucoma is and why the situation could be serious. We also usually want to achieve a certain outcome from the communication; in this case, you may want your father to agree to go to the ophthalmologist as soon as possible. Relaying information and getting something we want done may be vital to us, but we may not realize that the way in which we're communicating may be expressing complicated feelings about ourselves or the other person that we may not even be aware that we have.

Terms like "passive," "aggressive," and "assertive" are often used to describe the ways in which people communicate. Passive communication typically doesn't express what the person really means or wants. For example, your mother might say, "I can't take care of this house by myself anymore; I don't know what to do. It's too complicated for me to decide," and then be angry when you bring her brochures from an assisted living facility because what she really wanted you to do was to find her a cleaning service! Aggressive communication, in contrast, can directly express what someone wants, but in a way that is overly forceful and without consideration of the other person's feelings or desires. Your brother might say, for example, "Dad, you just have to go to the eye doctor, right away. There's no two ways about it, and that's that. We won't take no for an answer," only to discover that your father is so annoyed (and frightened) that he won't talk to him about the topic at all. Assertive communication is usually more helpful because it expresses directly what someone wants, too, but in a reasonable way that takes the needs and perspectives of others into account.

When you seem to be having trouble communicating with your relative, there are some points you might keep in mind:

- Try to step back and look at your own feelings and behavior. Your emotions and fears may be causing you to act or speak in a way that is disturbing or upsetting to your relative. Are you being aggressive and annoying? Passive and indirect? Check yourself out first!

- Make an effort to understand, in turn, if your relative's fears or feelings may be causing him or her to behave in a way that you view as unhelpful. If you think that is the case, try to keep your relative's perspective in mind as you talk and respond to his or her concerns—spoken or unspoken—sympathetically.

- Both you and your relative need emotional and perhaps other support during stressful times. Getting that kind of support can make everyone feel better and therefore possibly more able to work through challenging situations. In addition, if your relative has other family, friends, neighbors, current or former colleagues from work, and other trusted relationships with members of the clergy or medical profession, consider enlisting their aid in talking to him or her about some of the issues you are trying to resolve.

- Well-intentioned as you might be, however, sometimes you may not be the best person to talk to your relative about certain issues or about vision loss in general. Looking at how your family has handled stressful situations in the past can provide you with insight about whether you, a sibling, a close friend, or your clergyperson is best suited to discuss what is happening.

• Joining a family support group can be invaluable (see Chapters 5 and 9) as a way of discussing situations and getting insight into how to talk to your relative or deal with certain topics. Professional help, such as counseling or consultation with vision rehabilitation agency staff (see Chapters 1 and 5), is another resource that can make a difference.

Ultimately, everyone's life is his or her own, and this is true for your older relative. He or she is entitled to make life choices and decisions. You may not agree with something your relative does or does not do, and in such an instance, trying to be both patient and persistent, stepping back and then revisiting a topic later, may be the course of action to pursue with someone whose well-being matters to you.

HEARING LOSS AND ITS EFFECT ON COMMUNICATION

Communicating with your relative can become more complicated if he or she has experienced hearing loss as well as vision loss. Since approximately half the people aged 65 and older experience a loss in hearing, this may be a challenge you will need to face. A visual impairment may make tasks such as putting in a hearing aid or changing the batteries more difficult and discourage someone from using his or her aid. In such a case, your relative may misunderstand what you are saying or may not hear you at all, and his or her poor vision might make it more difficult to see your facial expressions as cues to what you're trying to say. Addressing the hearing loss may therefore be essential for good communication.

For this reason, it is important for you to understand exactly what your older relative can see and hear. If he or she displays signs of what you think may be paranoia, it may actually be the effects of impaired vision and hearing. Some older people with hearing loss may appear senile to others, simply because they cannot hear or see well. They may indeed become confused about what is going on, but not because of some neurological problem. All these factors may result in communication problems between you and your older relative, and more information about communicating with someone who has both vision and hearing losses is presented in Chapter 8, "Vision Loss and Other Health Conditions."

UNDERSTANDING THE DESIRE FOR INDEPENDENCE

Most people of any age want to live their own way, without having a different lifestyle imposed on them. And most people, regardless of age, do not want to be a burden to others, particularly to their children. At the same time that your older relative may be frightened and overwhelmed by what's happening, he or she may still wish to remain as independent as possible. It is important to respect this desire for independence, even if it makes you anxious about his or her well-being. Most older people have spent a lifetime pursuing their own goals, taking care of themselves and others, and meeting their responsibilities, and accepting help at this stage of their lives may be difficult for them. In addition to feeling ashamed of having to need or ask for help, they may often feel that by asking for help, they will sacrifice their independence, dignity, and control over their own lives. Consider the following scenario:

> *Mrs. Harrington has lived alone for several years since the death of her husband. She is diabetic, like many other African Americans. Although her husband had always helped her with her daily insulin shots, after his death she learned to inject the insulin herself and to do many other things around the house that her husband used to do. She is proud of herself for learning to cope so well.*
>
> *A few months ago, however, she noticed that her vision was blurring. She finally went for a checkup and found out that she had diabetic retinopathy. Laser surgery was not successful in one eye, and she has limited vision in the other eye. Her son James lives in another state and comes home monthly to visit.*
>
> *"Mom," James said to her on the phone the other day, "I won't take no for an answer. Sherri and I are just too worried*

about you all the time. Why, you can't even read the glucose meter when you test your blood sugar! You've simply got to sell the house and move in with us and the kids."

"I don't have to do anything. I can stay here, and I will," she replied, somewhat incensed at his tone. *"I can take care of myself just fine, James. Now, I know that the home health nurse who's helping me with the insulin shots will stop coming by soon. But she told me about a vision rehabilitation agency right here in town where I can learn how to do things better with my poor eyesight. Let me find out more about this before we make any hasty decisions."*

"Well, I guess that would be okay," James agreed. *"Why don't I go with you to the agency? I have some questions, too."*

You play a critical role in the life of your older relative who is experiencing vision loss. Your support is important to his or her adjustment, but knowing when to let go in the interest of your relative's need for self-determination is important too. Mrs. Harrington clearly wants to be independent, but she needs her son's encouragement and support in order to tackle this enormous task. She also needs to be able to maintain her dignity.

If you are finding it difficult to understand why your older relative may be being stubborn about refusing your assistance, try putting yourself in his or her shoes. Imagine how you might feel if you could no longer drive or take care of other everyday tasks that you take for granted. If you had lost the ability to control many aspects of your life, might you not want to keep control over the rest? When someone doesn't see well, it is natural to want to protect him or her, but natural protectiveness can prevent you from accepting your relative's need to make decisions for him- or herself.

You might want to ask, at this point, what kind of help can you provide without overwhelming your older relative? Help comes in many forms. If you use the "I-can-fix-it-for-you-Mom" model, all you would require from your mother would be for her to sit back and accept help. You could inundate her with assistance of all kinds and insist on doing everything for her. But this could send the message that you believe she cannot possibly learn how to care for herself. Chances are she doesn't want you to become her caregiver, and you don't want that either. Listen carefully to the feelings and concerns expressed by your older relative, and try to respond to them.

> "It is important to balance the roles that family members play in the lives of their older relatives: encourager, counselor, researcher, transporter, helper, advisor, confidant, companion, and caregiver."
>
> *–Dick N., San Francisco*

Rather than telling your mother what to do, it might be preferable to sit down with her and let her know that you are available to provide support and encourage-
ment and to be someone to count on while she's adjusting to the changes in her life. In general, don't overwhelm her (or yourself) by talking about your concerns all at one time. Go slowly. Bring up important topics in normal conversation, and suggest ideas and solutions as needs arise.[1] For example, if your mother tells you she missed a doctor's appointment because she couldn't see her clock, it might be the time to show her a catalogue that describes a large-numeral or talking clock. You can also take the opportunity to point out other items in the catalogue that may be of use to her or even to bring up the possibility of vision rehabilitation services.

Not every person who experiences vision loss feels passionately about staying independent, especially at first. Some people are overwhelmed and feel that they must now depend on others to do everything for them. They worry, "How can I possibly do anything for myself if I can't see?" It can be difficult to help people in such situations, but, as mentioned earlier in this chapter, sometimes you simply need to give them more time. You can seek the involvement of others, such as friends, family members, fellow church, synagogue, or mosque members, or counselors. The suggestions in Chapter 9 on getting support from friends and the community may help.

It is important to remember that the majority of older people with vision loss have some vision, and there are many ways to encourage independence. The adaptive techniques, low vision devices, vision rehabilitation services, and support groups described throughout this book can help your relative continue to live independently. It is also helpful to learn how to discuss and work out solutions in an ongoing way to the challenges that vision loss poses, as well as to your own fears about your older relative's living alone. (The suggestions about communication in this chapter may be helpful.) You may make it easier for your older relative to accept a degree of assistance by acknowledging his or her need for control and talking about how you can help without taking that control away. In some cases, it may also feel less threatening if you offer a reasonable amount of help—say, a ride to a medical appointment—rather than trying to take charge of everything at once.

INDEPENDENCE AND INTERDEPENDENCE: STRIKING A BALANCE

In our culture, we place a high value on independence. Building independence starts early in this country, as we prepare our children to take on the challenges of adulthood and rely on their parents less and less. For this and many other reasons, your relative may feel that being independent is critical and, conversely, may be frightened of no longer being able to take care of him- or herself. But sometimes the concept of *interdependence* is overlooked. Within this framework, people are helpful to each other, and it is natural to depend on others. For example, an older person might rely on younger relatives for assistance, while the younger relatives could also depend on the older person for child care, perhaps. No matter how independent your relative becomes in being able to carry out everyday tasks, situations may remain in which he or she will need to depend on someone, for example, when needing to be driven somewhere or having other access to transportation. Creating a situation where an individual doesn't just receive assistance, but also gives it, such as accepting deliveries when you're not home, may help that person maintain self-esteem and may make it easier for him or her to accept help in return.

When you begin to talk to a parent or other older relative about personal concerns, he or she may begin to feel the need to "give back" by offering you some kind of help or support. In some cases, being able to provide *you* with help will be important to your relative's adjustment process and continued psychological well-being, so don't turn down the offer. Perhaps you are going through a divorce and need to talk it over with someone you trust; perhaps your teenager is being rebellious and you need advice; perhaps you are having trouble with a coworker and are not sure how to handle the situation. Just because your relative has lost some vision doesn't mean that he or she isn't as insightful as before or cannot provide you with emotional support or good advice. Continuing to trust your relative's qualities as a human being is appropriate and can help him or her maintain self-esteem, self-confidence, and a feeling of independence at a difficult juncture in life.

REHABILITATION: YOUR CRITICAL ROLE

Unless your relative has other health conditions that limit the ability to live on his or her own, specialized rehabilitation services for people with visual impairments might make all the difference in helping him or her to continue an independent lifestyle. Agencies in most areas of the country provide instruction in adaptive techniques—either at the agency or right in your relative's home, as described in the next chapter. Vision rehabilitation therapists and orientation and mobility specialists can show your older relative how to carry out daily activities, move around the house safely, and even travel safely and independently. Not everyone with vision loss believes he or she can learn new techniques to achieve independence. However, a visit from one of these professionals, who can demonstrate how anyone can learn to do basic tasks, sometimes using only slightly different methods (as described

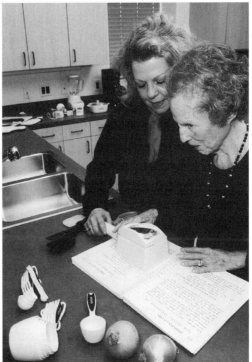

Earl Dotter

There are many ways for older people with vision loss to remain independent. You can play an important role by practicing vision rehabilitation skills at home with your older relative.

in Chapter 6), is often enough to motivate someone to want to learn more.

In some instances, family members can also take part in the instruction. Doing so can give you the chance to develop a better understanding of the skills your relative may be trying to develop and of how adaptive methods can enable him or her to carry out daily activities safely. You can play a significant role in vision rehabilitation of your relative by practicing the skills with him or her at home in between visits from the vision rehabilitation therapist. You can also help with organizing his or her house, under your relative's direction, to make it safer and easier to find everything (as described in Chapter 7). Or, if your relative is learning some cooking techniques, you might encourage him or her to cook something for a family meal. When you participate in the rehabilitation process, you might not only directly further your relative's movement toward independence, you might also prevent yourself from feeling helpless during what can be a difficult adjustment.

Finding the right way to introduce the subject of independent living and rehabilitation services may be difficult for you. There are different ways to introduce the concept and provide information on available resources. Raising issues indirectly may be a helpful strategy. For example, you might ask your father how he's keeping track of his pills since he has so many, and add that you can hardly keep track of your own. You can also watch for the openings that can arise for a discussion when your mother mentions the difficulty of writing a letter or cooking Thanksgiving dinner for the family. Talking in general terms about independent living issues may work for some people, while raising some specific examples might be more useful for others. Sometimes sharing your own emotions about your parent's vision loss might be persuasive. You might say, for example, "It bothers me so much to hear you say that you can't read any more. I remember you loved to read stories to me—reading is one of your great pleasures in life. You're missing out on church, and on your book club meetings too. Shouldn't we talk about this and what we can do to help you do things you like, but—maybe in a different way?"

Participating in a support group (discussed in Chapter 9) can help your older relative immensely. Other people who have had to deal with the same issues and who have accomplished similar goals can provide affirmation to someone's feelings as well as encouragement and a great deal of useful information. Your relative may end up learning and understanding more about dealing with vision loss, and he or she may be able to give you new insights about it as well.

Sometimes people need professional counseling to adjust to vision loss and achieve an outlook that helps them continue an independent lifestyle. It is not uncommon for the whole family to go through this process—either together or individually. Overall, professional counselors can help make adjustment smoother for everyone.

You may find that you need to help your relative find vision rehabilitation services and additional help such as support groups in the area. Be prepared to help or look for sources of help if he or she asks you to do so. Once you've located them, the decision to use them should be left to your relative. If you feel that time passes and your relative needs help but is not doing anything about seeking it, you may need to make contact with rehabilitation professionals yourself and consult with them.

The support older people receive from family members while they are adjusting to vision loss is critical, as a number of studies have shown.[2] More than anything else, emotional support can help your older relative adapt to vision loss, overcome depression, and become satisfied with life.[3] Research has shown that family members can ease the adjustment to vision loss by listening to their relatives' feelings and offering help when it's needed.[4] Family and friends can play a key role by providing understanding and encouragement without pressure as your relative works through various issues and changes in his or her life. Your relative needs time to come to terms with vision loss and to consider engaging in the process of maintain his or her own life.

Chapter 5

Finding Professional Help

Ever since his parents had passed away five years ago, Bill had grown closer to his Aunt Franny and Uncle Tony, who had no children of their own. When Tony, at age 77, lost much of his vision to age-related macular degeneration, Bill took an active role in helping his aunt and uncle deal with the situation.

"I don't want to just sit around like a bump on a log," Tony told Bill after they got back from the ophthalmologist's office. "You know me. I need to keep busy. But how am I going to get to the senior center now? How can I play cards with the guys if I can't see the numbers? And they have a class there on how to use a computer to check on my investments. Forget that! I just don't know where to start. Everything I used to do without even thinking is almost impossible for me to handle now. I don't even know how to dial a phone number anymore."

Bill listened, but he didn't have any answers. Later that evening, he did some research on the Internet and discovered that there was an agency nearby that offered a wide variety of vision rehabilitation services for older people. He called first thing in the morning and found out that his uncle could set up an appointment soon. In the meantime, the representative from the agency suggested that Tony and his family attend a support group for older people experiencing vision loss.

That night, Bill showed up at his aunt and uncle's house with a big smile on his face. "I think I know what our next step is, Uncle Tony, and I think you're going to like it."

When people experience vision loss, they may not be aware that help is available to them. Every state has agencies that are staffed by experts who provide specialized services to help people learn how to live life after vision loss. Surprisingly, many eye care professionals are not aware of these services either, and therefore may not put their patients in touch with them. Medical professionals such as ophthalmologists focus on treating disease through medicine and surgery, but may know very little about services that help people live with vision loss that can't be corrected by these methods. This state of affairs stems in part from the often-fragmented nature of health care across the United States. In addition, because vision rehabilitation services are not covered by Medicare or by most insurance plans, they are outside the mainstream of the health care system. This situation may be changing, however, as more and more people become aware of how many older people are experiencing vision problems, particularly macular degeneration, and seek solutions.

Nevertheless, services that can provide critical guidance and support for you and your older relative do exist, and they can be obtained through vision rehabilitation agencies. There are both state and private organizations that provide a range of assistance designed to help people make the most effective use of their remaining vision.

A QUICK WAY TO find a vision rehabilitation agency in your community is by contacting organizations listed in the Resources section of this book, such as the American Foundation for the Blind (AFB), which publishes a directory of agencies throughout the U.S. and Canada. It also has an online search at www.afb.org/services.asp.

WHAT IS VISION REHABILITATION?

Vision rehabilitation is a combination of specialized training and counseling services that can help your older relative develop the special skills and techniques necessary to engage in day-to-day activities with vision loss. Vision rehabilitation cannot restore vision, but it can restore the ability of older people who have lost their vision to function in everyday life and regain their independence. Vision rehabilitation includes *orientation and mobility* instruction, *low vision therapy,* and *vision rehabilitation therapy* (also known as rehabilitation teaching or independent living skills instruction). Older individuals are also eligible for *vocational rehabilitation* services, typically after they receive training in independent living skills, to allow them to remain or become employed.

"When I first began to experience a vision loss it was frustrating and overwhelming to cope and to try to find information about what to do next. I went from place to place trying to find help and answers to my questions. I can visualize this vision rehabilitation center as being the light at the end of the tunnel."

–Harold S., Dallas

Not only can vision rehabilitation offer critical skills for someone who is living with vision loss, it can also help that person gain self-confidence. The daughter of a woman who lost her vision wrote, "It's very helpful for my mom to go to a vision rehabilitation agency and learn there are others out there with low vision who are living their lives successfully. She's been inspired to want to do more for herself." Most likely, your older relative will benefit just as much.

WHO ARE THE REHABILITATION PROFESSIONALS?

There are several types of professionals involved in vision rehabilitation, including vision rehabilitation therapists, low vision therapists, orientation and mobility specialists, occupational therapists, and vocational rehabilitation counselors. You and your older relative will probably meet many or all of them throughout the rehabilitation process.

VISION REHABILITATION THERAPISTS

The vision rehabilitation therapist, or rehabilitation teacher, is usually the first professional your older relative will work with once he or she is receiving services from a vision rehabilitation agency. Your older relative will learn to use his or her remaining vision or other senses, such as touch, to do routine daily tasks—everything you typically do around the house from morning until bedtime. This could include cooking or making coffee, reading the newspaper or mail with magnification, using special handwriting aids for correspondence, identifying and matching clothing in the closet, taking and keeping track of medication, and managing a checkbook. (Many of these basic techniques are explained in Chapter 6.) Besides this training in independent living skills, the vision rehabilitation therapist can offer training in the use of devices that help with these tasks (such as a signature guide or liquid level indicator for pouring, also discussed in Chapter 6), instruction in braille if that will be useful for taking notes or jotting down telephone numbers, and moving around safely indoors. Your older relative may also learn to use special computer technology or a closed-circuit television (CCTV) that magnifies materials and projects them onto a screen.

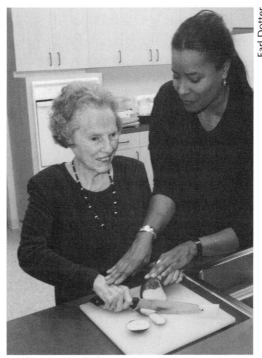

The vision rehabilitation therapist starts by assessing the client's ability to carry out various everyday activities, such as those involved in cooking, eating, dressing, bathing, doing laundry, and so forth. Typically this is done simply by asking how the individual does the

The vision rehabilitation therapist constructs a plan of instruction in daily living skills, such as cooking, that is tailored to your older relative's needs.

task, but sometimes the vision rehabilitation therapist will request that the older person demonstrate an action, such as pouring a cold liquid. The vision rehabilitation therapist can then construct a plan of instruction tailored to your older relative's needs.

Many vision rehabilitation therapists receive university training at the master's level and may receive certification as well, while some are trained by their agency. You may also encounter vision rehabilitation therapist assistants who assist vision rehabilitation therapists in teaching skills, but do not do assessments.

LOW VISION THERAPISTS

Low vision therapist is a new professional discipline in the vision field. Low vision therapists are certified, and they are therefore referred to as "certified low vision therapists" (CLVTs). They teach people how to use the special optical devices prescribed by the low vision specialist (either an optometrist or ophthalmologist with special training in low vision, as described in Chapter 2). These devices can include handheld magnifiers (some of which have built-in lights), telescopic lenses for distance viewing, high-intensity lighting, and magnifying lenses mounted in frames. Electronic devices such as computers with large-print or speech output and the closed-circuit television for reading fall into this category as well.

You might be wondering why someone would need training in the use of a magnifier. Using a magnifier is not as easy as it looks! Your older relative needs to learn the correct distance to maintain between the reading material or object and the device to keep the material in focus and make the best use of the magnifier without getting too fatigued. The low vision therapist will be able to teach your older relative with low vision how to use the magnifier and all of these other devices.

ORIENTATION AND MOBILITY SPECIALISTS

The orientation and mobility (O&M) specialist assesses and teaches travel skills. *Orientation* refers to the ability to know where one is in the surrounding environment and what objects or obstacles are present, and *mobility* refers to the ability to move safely and independently on one's own within that environment. Typically, O&M specialists will ask their clients where they usually want or need to go and then will develop a plan to teach them how to get there. There are also O&M assistants who work only under the supervision of O&M specialists because of the significant safety issues involved in teaching someone how to travel.

O&M specialists can teach independent travel skills, including using a sighted guide (that is, how to walk while being guided by another person, sometimes referred to as "human guide," which is described in Chapter 6), mastering self-protective techniques, using a long white cane, and traveling on public transportation. Because of their special training, they are qualified to teach people to travel outdoors as well as inside. Individuals learn to use auditory cues and their remaining vision to travel around the home and neighborhood—and even beyond. For example, your older relative can learn to use a white cane in order to get to the mailbox, the grocery store, or place of worship depending on his or her interest and proficiency. Uncle Tony, whom you met at the beginning of this chapter, can learn to use the bus to get to the senior center or to visit a friend. (And, in Chapter 6 you can find out how he can continue to use his computer and in Chapter 10, how he can keep playing cards with his buddies.)

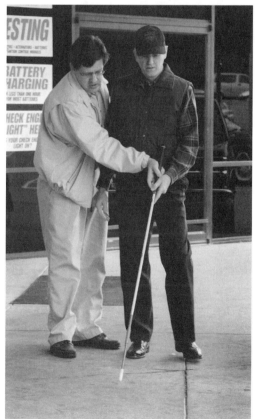

O&M specialists do not teach people how to work with a dog guide. (Dog guide is the generic term for dogs that are trained to guide people who are blind.) There are special schools for learning to work with a dog. Interested individuals have to apply to a school and must be capable of adequately caring for and exercising a dog. The training program typically takes at least a month and must be done at one of various residential schools around the country. (These schools are listed in the *AFB*

O&M specialists can teach a variety of independent travel skills, including how to use a long white cane to get around safely outdoors.

Directory of Services mentioned earlier; see the Resources section for more information.)

OCCUPATIONAL THERAPISTS

Occupational therapists have not traditionally been part of the vision rehabilitation field, but in their work with people with other disabilities they often encounter people with vision problems. Many have obtained training in low vision so they can help their patients experiencing vision loss, although they are not typically trained to work with people who are totally blind. Occupational therapists have training in working with people on independent living skills, but usually not in the same specialized manner as the vision rehabilitation therapist. As the number of low vision training programs has increased during the last decade, some private vision rehabilitation agencies have begun to hire occupational therapists, who have historically been part of the medical system and are therefore reimbursable by Medicare. There are also occupational therapist assistants.

VOCATIONAL REHABILITATION COUNSELORS

The focus of vocational rehabilitation counselors who work with people who have visual impairments is to consider whether they are good candidates for employment and help them to find jobs when they are ready. Older persons with vision loss often feel they can no longer work, particularly before they have achieved some success in independent living. Vocational rehabilitation counselors can encourage them to consider the possibility of employment. The counselor develops an employment plan in conjunction with the older person, assists with job

"I had a background in management, but I never thought I'd be able to keep working once I started to lose my sight when I was 67. The vocational counselor worked with me to develop a business plan and provided the seed money to start my own business providing medical identification cards."

—Luis H., Orlando

placement, and provides the necessary services and equipment to make work possible for a person with visual impairment.

Vocational rehabilitation counselors have recently begun to witness an increasing number of older people seeking employment—because they need additional funds, are bored at home, or just want to be engaged in something productive. The vision rehabilitation therapist, orientation and mobility specialist, low vision therapist, and vocational rehabilitation counselor often work as a team with a social worker or case manager from an agency to make sure that their clients receive all the necessary comprehensive services, including employment.

SUPPORT GROUPS

Becoming involved in a support group may be the most helpful and important thing that either you or your older relative can do for yourselves. Many agencies provide support groups for older people who are newly visually impaired and also for their relatives. A staff member such as a social worker sometimes leads a group, although frequently an older person with vision loss who has successfully completed a vision rehabilitation program may do so as well. If your older relative is someone who enjoys taking on new challenges and roles, he or she might look forward to serving as a support group facilitator for his or her peers after receiving vision rehabilitation services. Often, older people say that of all the help and training they received, their support group had the greatest impact. The benefit of having the opportunity to meet others who talk about their eye conditions and, even more important, share their concerns, frustrations, and process of adjustment, cannot be underestimated.

In some communities where the vision rehabilitation agency has a waiting list for services, the agency organizes a support group so that people can have this meaningful experience while they are awaiting training. Families are usually relieved to know that their older relatives have the opportunity to make this connection. Agencies have also started groups for individuals who have completed training that provide ongoing support for individuals who may enjoy the contact and the opportunity to help others who are losing vision.

In addition to your local vision rehabilitation agency you can find information about support groups in *Sharing Solutions*, a newsletter published by Lighthouse International for people with vision loss and their support networks. Lighthouse International also maintains a national directory of over 4,000 existing support groups. In addition, there are two large national organizations of individuals who are blind or visually impaired—the American Council of the Blind and the National Federation of the Blind—that have local chapters throughout the country and are a good source of support and information. (See the Resources section in the back of this book for contact information for all these organizations.)

Older people who are experiencing vision loss and their families may start a support group if one does not exist in their area. This happens more frequently when people live in retirement facilities or in senior citizen apartment buildings, which eliminates the need for transportation to the group. In most cases, individuals initiate the idea with the staff at their vision rehabilitation agency, who then help with the necessary arrangements.

It's possible that you or your older relative may need more assistance with adjustment to vision loss beyond a support group. There may be a professional on staff at the vision rehabilitation agency who can provide individual counseling. If not, your relative's vision rehabilitation professional can help connect you and your older relative to counseling assistance.

SUPPORT FOR THE SUPPORTERS

As has been mentioned throughout this handbook, you and other family members will also need support during your older relative's adjustment to vision loss. Everyone's emotions can run high during this process. You might be finding it difficult at this point to imagine how the situation could improve or return to some level of normalcy and might benefit the most from accurate information about what to expect and what is possible, as well as learning some coping strategies.

Once you are connected to a vision rehabilitation agency, you will find it important to ask about services for families. Many agencies sponsor open-house sessions for family members through which they can acquire accurate information about the issues just mentioned. Some invite family members for a family day or to participate in part of the vision rehabilitation program. There, you can see firsthand that your older relative is able to learn adaptive skills and to function safely.

You may also benefit tremendously from participating in a support group solely for family members, where you can share information and coping strategies with others. Learning that your family is not the only one struggling with the onset of vision loss can help you a great deal through the adjustment process. Not all agencies have support groups for family members, but be sure to inquire if one is not mentioned. (This topic is discussed further in Chapter 9.)

SUCCESS STORIES

The following stories demonstrate the dramatic difference that vision rehabilitation services can make in the lives of older persons and their families. In these real-life circumstances, shared by vision rehabilitation staff throughout the country, professionals introduce you to older people with vision loss and describe the kinds of services they received to help them continue to function independently and to enjoy life. Some of the stories mention specific types of devices and equipment used in the rehabilitation process that will be discussed in Chapter 6.

HUGH K. IN MISSISSIPPI

Hugh K. is 88 years old. His daughter referred him to the independent living program when he was diagnosed with age-related macular degeneration. Retired from the U.S. Air Force, he served in WWII and the Korean Conflict. Afterward, he returned to Mississippi, where he was the Executive Director of the Mississippi Manufacturers Association (MMA). In this position he lobbied not only the state legislature but also the U.S. Congress to bring quality companies and manufacturing jobs to the state. After his retirement from MMA, he continued to work part-time as a lobbyist, continuing to bring jobs and manufacturing to Mississippi. Very active in the work world, he was also an avid golf and bridge player.

When his vision began to fail, he found working difficult, as reading contracts and handling correspondence was almost impossible. Golf became difficult and bridge was no longer enjoyable. At this time, he felt it best to retire. However, he was extremely unhappy just sitting at home and being unable to continue with his hobbies. He and his family began looking for resources that would enable him to "find something to do" and help him regain his independence.

His daughter contacted the vision rehabilitation agency in the community after hearing about it from another older person who had gotten services there. Services provided by the vision rehabilitation therapist included training with low vision assistive technology (such as a computer with speech output), help with personal adjustment, peer-support groups, provision of low vision devices, instruction in adapted ways to carry out routine daily activities, and information and referral services.

Since receiving these services and equipment, Ryan's whole world has changed. He has written a book on his role in the Korean Conflict, was instrumental in establishing the Mississippi National Guard Museum at Camp Shelby, has worn out numerous decks of low vision bridge cards, has learned to enjoy his golfing friends on and off the course, and has been called upon to speak to the Mississippi legislature regarding future funding for the Mississippi Department of Rehabilitation Services.

OTIS T. IN FLORIDA

Otis T., age 81, was helped by a vocational rehabilitation counselor to become self-employed as a tax accountant working out of his home. He has been earning $1,500 a month. Although Mr. T. was already retired from a successful career, he was able to learn how to use access technology, such as speech access with his computer, to complete tax returns.

Through the specialized services available from vision rehabilitation professionals, older people experiencing vision loss can accomplish almost any goal they might have—including learning to take care of their daily needs, traveling, enjoying leisure activities, or even working. As you can see from the real-life accounts in this chapter, learning new skills and attaining independence are within reach for your older relative. Encouraging him or her to start on the road to independence by getting involved with a vision rehabilitation agency, a support group, and even employment counseling can begin to make all the difference. As you and your older relative take these momentous first steps, remember: Many others have succeeded before you, and a wide variety of resources and trained professionals are there to support you through the adjustment process.

Chapter 6

A New Approach to Everyday Tasks

Cindy dropped off her mother, Ann, at the bank, as she has done each month since her mother lost much of her vision to glaucoma several years ago.

"Do you need any help, Mom?"

"No," her mother replied, "I'll be fine. You'll park in the usual spot, right?"

"Of course."

Carefully but assuredly, Ann stepped out of the car. She listened for other people on the sidewalk, and then placed her long white cane in front of her to check for obstacles, just as the O&M specialist at the rehabilitation agency had showed her.

When she got inside, she pulled out her Social Security check, along with a little plastic writing guide, and casually asked the teller to show her where she needed to sign.

"I'd like $100 in cash back from the deposit—four twenties and two ten-dollar bills, please," she told the teller. "And could you hand them to me separately please, so I know which is which?"

"Not a problem."

Many family members make the assumption that vision loss will prevent an older relative from cooking, handling a checking account, doing laundry, or managing any number of other daily tasks. On the contrary: Through the use of adaptive methods discussed in this chapter, as well as some specialized equipment, your older relative can carry out most tasks that he or she may wish or need to do. Some of the techniques described in this chapter will give you ideas about how you can help your older relative gain the information, confidence, and skills to do many activities efficiently and independently.

Keep in mind that some people want to start learning right away, while others may take a while to adjust to the onset of vision loss before they take steps forward. In the latter case you can help your older relative by being patient and empathetic. Adjusting to vision loss takes time for both of you, as do working out ways to interact and communicate with each other. Also, you may not feel comfortable taking on the role of instructor and may wish to seek professional assistance from a vision rehabilitation agency such as those described in Chapter 5.

If your older relative prefers to learn things on his or her own, or if there is a waiting list at your local vision rehabilitation agency, instructional materials are available that can help you and your older relative get started. They are also good for reinforcing information learned through an agency. Hadley School for the Blind

"Special training has given me back my freedom and my independence. I am once again a responsible adult making my own decisions and living my own life. Losing one's sight is not the end of one's existence. You simply need to relearn how to do basic tasks with a few adaptations."
—*Dr. Margaret C., San Antonio*

has a long-standing reputation in developing free correspondence courses on tape—and now online—about basic topics involving age-related vision loss. VISIONS Services for the Blind and Visually Impaired, a private vision rehabilitation agency, has several sets of cassettes available for sale to the public for teaching oneself adaptive techniques. (See the Resources section for contact information.)

Books that might help you are also available. One useful book is *Making Life More Livable*, which describes many of these adaptive techniques in even further detail. If you prefer more structured instruction with information provided in a lesson format, check out *Solutions for Success*. If you would rather watch a video that describes adaptive skills, take a look at *Solutions for Everyday Living for Older People with Visual Impairments*. All these resources are available through AFB Press, and more information about these, as well as other sources of information, can be found in the Resources section.

The following sections present some tasks your older relative may be interested in mastering using adaptive techniques or equipment. The tasks included are basic activities that many older people feel they may still be able to do and will want to do in order to remain independent. Unless otherwise indicated, the alternative methods discussed here are ones you and your older relative can work on together even before going to a vision rehabilitation agency. Your older relative can also practice these skills between training sessions provided by the agency.

You may find yourself taking on many different roles with your older relative in regard to learning these new skills—instructing, reinforcing, supporting, facilitating, or a combination. If your older relative has already received vision rehabilitation services and learned some of these techniques from a vision rehabilitation therapist, you may be in a position to reinforce the skills, especially if you participated in the teaching sessions and have an understanding of the adaptive methods and how they work best for him or her.

As you continue reading, please keep this in mind: *Do not take over tasks for your older relative who is experiencing vision loss.* This can damage his or her self-esteem and slow down the process of learning new skills. Help your older relative to continue to live as independently (or interdependently) as possible by asking before providing assistance and helping when requested.

BASIC TECHNIQUES FOR ADAPTATION

Certain basic techniques are fundamental when adapting tasks and the everyday environment for a person with vision loss. These include

- organizing meticulously
- labeling
- using tactile markers and devices
- using contrast and color
- creating environmental cues

ORGANIZING

One of the most important aspects of adapting daily tasks so that they can be done by someone with vision loss is the need for organization. Organization means having a particular place for things and keeping them in their place. If items are not where they are expected to be, people with vision loss have trouble finding them. Many of us have the habit of absentmindedly setting down a pair of reading glasses and then forgetting where we left them. But if your uncle has low vision, he cannot quickly, or even slowly, scan the environment to locate his misplaced lenses. Often, when an important item is misplaced, an older person can actually start to panic about locating it. Therefore, one of the first habits your older relative should develop is keeping things in their designated place, and it is equally important for you to do the same.

LABELING

Labeling items in a way that makes sense is another good technique. For example, cans of food tend to look pretty similar, so labeling them in a way that your older relative can easily recognize is important. Labeling clothes according to their color is also important, since your older relative may no longer be able to recognize which shirt matches which pair of pants.

TACTILE MARKERS AND DEVICES

Markers that can be easily felt, also known as tactile indicators, are one form of labeling. For example, marking the temperature

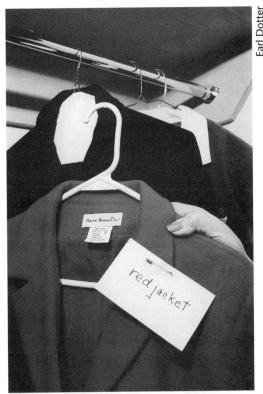

Earl Dotter

Labeling items for easy recognition is one of the key techniques for adapting everyday activities.

settings on the stove or washing machine using a substance called Hi-Marks to make raised dots is an effective way to help your older relative use these appliances. Tactile markers can even be placed on the TV remote control to distinguish channel, volume, and power buttons. There are also many products and devices available for purchase that make use of markings that can be felt. For example, paper with raised lines can be helpful when writing a letter, and tactile rulers have raised marks at the designated intervals.

CONTRAST AND COLOR

The use of contrast—both in brightness and color—is an effective way to make text or objects more visible for older individuals with low vision. It is useful for reading, labeling, signs, table settings, and even the color scheme in the home. You will have to determine which type of contrast works best for your older relative. For example, some individuals see dark colors on a light background better than light on dark. Keep in mind that older people generally find it easier to see darker, more saturated colors than pastels, and two pastel colors together are virtually impossible to distinguish.

ENVIRONMENTAL CUES

Environmental cues refer to objects or other sensory stimuli in the environment (such as sounds or odors) that help an individual identify his or her location and get oriented. Environmental cues and techniques are covered in the next chapter.

ALTERNATIVE METHODS FOR DAILY TASKS

The basic techniques just described are referred to often in the tips for adapting everyday tasks that follow. The special adapted products mentioned throughout can be found in the independent living catalogs listed in the Resources section.

COOKING

Here are a few basic strategies that can make working in the kitchen and cooking a safe and satisfying activity for your older relative:

- **Organize foods in closets and cabinets in a way that is useful and makes sense to your older relative.** For example, keep frequently used items in the front of the cabinet, or place ingredients for dishes that are made often next to each other in the cabinet. Organizing foods and cooking utensils in related groups according to areas of activity in the kitchen can be very helpful as well. You might want to help by making suggestions, but, ultimately, let your older relative make the decisions.

- **Label items, such as cans of food, with your older relative's own system of marking.** For a person with low vision who can see large print, you and your older relative can cover the existing label and write the name of the contents with a thick, dark felt-tip pen or marker. (A good pen for this purpose, called "20/20," can be found in independent living catalogs, along with other products for labeling.) Another labeling system consists of miniature food items made out of plastic, which can be attached to cans. Some people use a system of rubber bands to indicate the contents of a can; for example, one rubber band might mean chicken soup, two rubber bands for vegetable soup, and so forth.

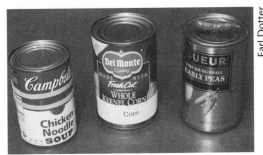

There are a variety of labeling systems that you and your older relative can try to find the one that works best.

- **Mark appliances and equipment with a product that will make a raised mark to indicate various settings.** For example, you can use Hi-Marks to mark the stove, microwave, and other appliances, so that your older relative can locate settings either visually or tactilely. It is not helpful to mark *every* setting,

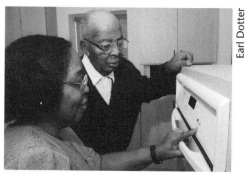
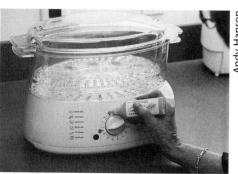

Earl Dotter

Andy Hanson

Marking appliances with a product that leaves a raised mark helps someone with vision loss to locate frequently used settings.

however. Label the temperatures used most fre-quently, such as 350 degrees on the oven dial, or "one minute" and "start" on the microwave. This technique works for thermostats, the washer and dryer, and other appliances as well.

- **Pay attention to lighting in the kitchen.** Having enough light to see what one is doing is critical in the kitchen. Good lighting is also safer, since using sharp cooking knives can be dangerous in dim light. First, maintain good overall lighting in the kitchen by having a strong ceiling light. You might also want to install good task lighting, or light directly over the areas where you work in the kitchen. Good examples of where task lighting is needed most are over the stove and over the cutting board. (Lighting is dis-cussed in more detail in Chapter 7.)
- **Remind your older relative not to wear long sleeves while cooking.** They can catch on fire easily, particularly when reaching for the pots on the back burners of gas stoves.
- **Look in independent living catalogs for adaptive versions of kitchen equipment that your older rel-ative commonly uses.** Examples include large-print or raised-line measuring cups, large-print measuring spoons, long oven mitts that cover the arms, a tomato slicer, kitchen timers with large-print or raised-print markings, special safety food turners, both dark and light cutting boards to provide con-

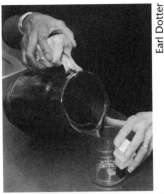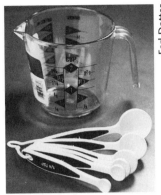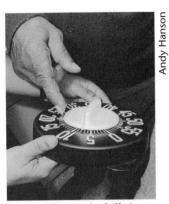

A liquid level indicator (left), which beeps when a cup or glass is nearly full, is especially useful for pouring hot liquids. Some other useful items in the kitchen are these measuring cups and spoons (center) and timer (right), all with large, contrasting print.

trast with different foods and make it easier to see what is being cut, and liquid level indicators for pouring liquids. The liquid level indicator is a particularly interesting and useful device. When placed on the rim of a cup or glass, it beeps when the vessel is nearly full so that the pourer knows to stop before the liquid overflows. It is particularly useful for pouring hot liquids, which can be dangerous.

- **Reinforce what your older relative has learned during independent living skills training.** Remind your older relative how to use the adaptive equipment and how to operate appliances with the new markings.
- **Instill good safety habits in the kitchen.** Remind your older relative to always close cabinet doors after opening them, turn pot handles over the stove, and wipe up spills on the floor immediately after they occur. Make sure you check for frayed electrical cords and throw away expired products as well.

EATING

The most important aspect of eating is helping your older relative know how to locate his or her plate and the food on it, as well as utensils and beverages at the table.

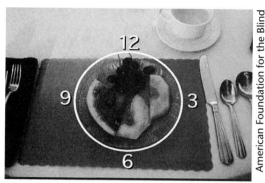

The clock method is an excellent way to describe the location of food on a plate and items in a place setting.

- **The clock method is an excellent way to describe the location of food on the plate and items in the place setting.** Mentally superimpose the face of a clock on the plate and use the numbers to indicate where the items are placed. For example, you can tell your dad that his roast beef is at noon on his plate and his water glass at 2:00 in his place setting.

- **Use contrast for the place setting to help your older relative locate the plate and other items at the table.** For instance, you could use a brightly colored placemat on top of a white tablecloth and under a white plate. Drinking glasses that provide contrast with the beverage that is in them are also preferable, such as a white coffee cup to contrast with the dark coffee.

- **Place the plate on a nonskid, contrasting surface, such as piece of cloth shelf liner.** This material comes in different colors, can be cut to fit the situation, and is washable.

- **Specialized utensils might be helpful.** Options include a rocker knife that has a T-shaped handle to fit

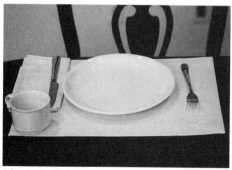
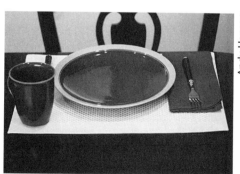

Placing dishes on a contrasting place mat (right) makes them much easier to see than white dishes on a white mat (left).

the hand and is easy to use for people who have a weak grasp; a plastic bumper guard that fits around a plate so that the food does not fall off; and an audible liquid level indicator that beeps when you have nearly filled a cup. Although many of these adaptive eating items have been developed for people with physical disabilities, they are also use-

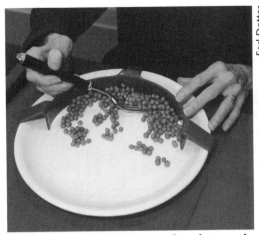

A bumper guard fits around a plate and keeps food from falling off.

ful for those who are visually impaired.

Your older relative's vision rehabilitation therapist will demonstrate other specific techniques and devices as well, such as tips for cutting food. (More detailed information on eating techniques is available in the books and videos listed in the Resource section.)

WRITING

Many different types of writing devices exist that can help your older relative with tasks such as signing his or her name on a check or addressing an envelope legibly. Some examples are letter-writing guides, signature guides, check-writing templates, envelope-writing guides, bold-line and raised-line paper, and bold-line pens, all of which are available through vision rehabilitation agencies and specialty products catalogues.

A signature guide is a small piece of plastic or cardboard with a space cut out in the middle for someone experiencing vision loss to write his or her signature. The person with vision loss can ask a merchant or other person requiring his or her signature to place the opening of the signature guide on the signature line of a document or credit card slip. The development of the signature guide made a big difference in making obsolete the antiquated method of asking a blind people to make an X for their signature! These are very inexpensive items; the signature guide only costs about $1.00. The check-writing guide,

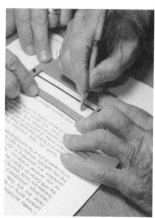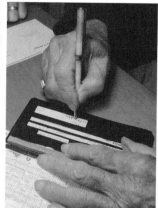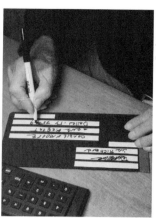

Earl Dotter

The signature guide (left), check-writing guide (center), and envelope-addressing template (right) are all helpful writing guides.

letter-writing guide, and envelope-addressing templates are similar, with openings in the places where the necessary information is written. These devices are relatively simple in design, but they do require practice. Your older relative will need to try out different types to determine which are the most useful and easiest to use. You can assist in practice by placing the openings over the spaces where information needs to be provided. Continue to work with your older relative until he or she feels secure about filling in the information.

Placing writing aids on a contrasting surface may help your older relative see where to write. These guides are frequently black or another dark color, since they are typically used with white paper. They would not work as well for addressing a red envelope, for example, due to lack of contrast between the guide, the envelope, and the ink.

Bold-line paper provides darker lines and larger spaces between each line. Raised-line paper is similar, only the bold lines are also raised. These types of paper make it easier to write a letter or make a shopping list.

USING A COMPUTER

Using a computer to write and communicate may appeal to your older relative. Recent models come equipped with screen magnification programs that can enlarge the print appearing on the computer monitor display. Magnification levels are measured in power levels, such as 2× (2 power, or print twice as large as normal) and go as high as 16× magnification. However, the larger the magnification your older relative needs, the smaller the viewing area, or the amount of text that can be seen on the screen. This is often difficult for the older person to adjust to because he or she wants to be able to read the screen in the same way he or she did prior to vision loss. Your older relative will have to learn to be patient with seeing a small piece of information at a time. You can assist by helping him or her understand that this is how the equipment works and that it is not his or her limitations that make the process slower than before.

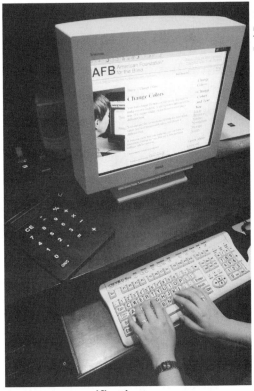

Earl Dotter

A screen magnification program can make a computer usable for someone with low vision. This keyboard also has large-print keys.

Many people with impaired vision use special screen reader software that can read aloud the text that is displayed on the computer monitor in a synthetic voice. The voice can be changed to meet the needs of the user. For example, some individuals find it easier to understand a male than a female voice due to the lower pitch. The reading speed can also be changed. Screen readers not only read aloud text within a document, but also information within dialog boxes and error messages. Screen readers can read aloud menu options and the labels for graphical icons on the desktop. Recent upgrades have made the use of the Internet easier as well.

Some software applications have features that include screen magnification and a screen reader. You and your older relative can ask your vision rehabilitation therapist more about these and other types of software and equipment and their functions. (If you're interested in learning more about this type of assistive technology for people with vision loss, there are a number of places to look on the Internet, including the assistive technology section of the American Foundation for the Blind's Web site at www.afb.org.)

READING MAIL

Reading mail and bills often presents a major challenge for an older person with vision loss. There are several options available, depending on one's level of vision. Some of these include low vision devices such as magnifiers or closed-circuit television systems, which are discussed in greater depth in Chapter 10. An optical character recognition (OCR) system is an option for individuals with limited vision. These can be either stand-alone machines or computer applications that use a flatbed scanner and software to read aloud printed text. Relying on a personal reader—a friend or someone hired for a few hours a week—may be an option, if your older relative feels comfortable with this solution. Items could even be faxed to a family member to be read.

BANKING AND WRITING CHECKS

Being able to handle one's own finances is a large part of independence, and for this reason you'll want to make it possible for your older relative to manage his or her bank account. Large-print and raised-line checks are available from most banks; simply inquire about them at your older relative's branch. If his or her bank does not carry them, they can be ordered through one of the catalogs listed in the Resources section. Here are a few other tips for banking:

- **Large-print check registers are available through catalogs or can be set up on a computer.**
- **Banks are required to make statements available in large print, braille, or on cassette, if requested.** Today, most banks also offer online banking. If your older relative feels comfortable using a computer,

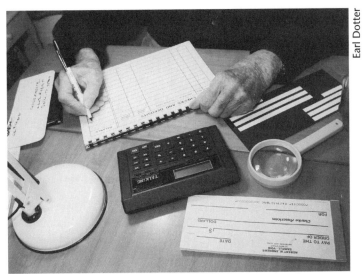

Large-print check registers and checks and a talking calculator can all help an older person with vision loss manage finances independently.

this can be an excellent alternative to managing print and paper. The vision rehabilitation therapist can assist with developing these skills. Also, certain bills such as utilities can be deducted automatically from a checking account, eliminating the need for writing a check.

- **Check-writing guides, described in the section on writing, make writing checks easier.**
- **Low vision and "talking" calculators are available for balancing checkbooks and statements.** (Talking devices are described in a later section.)

See the next section for suggestions on how your older relative can identify his or her money when getting cash from the bank.

IDENTIFYING MONEY

Money identification is an easy task to manage once your older relative knows a few basic tips. You can help. Suggest that your older relative use a wallet that has four or more compartments for paper money so that bills can be sorted easily. When not

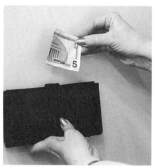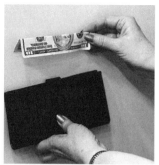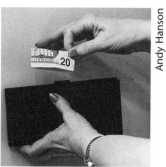

Andy Hanson

A system of folding bills of different denominations in different ways helps to identify money.

using a multi-compartment wallet, bills can be folded in different ways to differentiate among them:

- Keep one-dollar bills unfolded and extended flat.
- Fold five-dollar bills in half with the short ends together.
- Fold ten-dollar bills in half lengthwise with the long sides together.
- Fold twenty-dollar bills in half and then fold in half again.

Your older relative can ask merchants and cashiers to list the denominations of paper money they are handing to him or her and then can fold the bills in a manner described. You may need to practice the money management system with your older relative and encourage him or her to ask for help with identifying bills. Electronic bill identifiers are available through the catalogs but are relatively expensive.

Coins can be identified by size and touch. Pennies and nickels have smooth sides; dimes and quarters have rough edges. Dollar coins have smooth edges. Once your older relative has learned these cues, he or she can practice them with you before using this newly acquired skill in public.

USING THE TELEPHONE

Most telephones today are the push-button style, and with practice your older relative can learn to dial by memorizing the positions of the numbers. The left column has numbers 1, 4, 7; the middle has 2, 5, 8, 0 and the right column has 3, 6, and 9. On most American-made phones, the number 5 has a tactile marking. The 4, 5, and 6 keys are considered the "home row," where the fingers can rest, just like the home row on a computer keyboard. From those keys, the other number keys can be found by moving one row up or down. Small colored touch dots can be used to identify these keys as well.

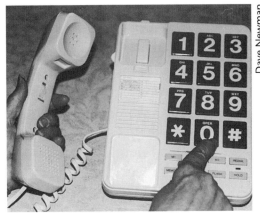

A pushbutton telephone with large numerals makes dialing easy.

Some telephones are made with large-print numbers and buttons with contrasting colors. These may be useful if your older relative has low vision and can see the large numbers. Another option is to purchase a programmable phone into which frequently used numbers can be programmed. Using this type of phone, one normally has to dial only one or two numbers. Voice-recognition phones that dial a number when a person's name or other word is spoken are another option, but you would need to test such a phone with your older relative's voice to ensure that it is reliable.

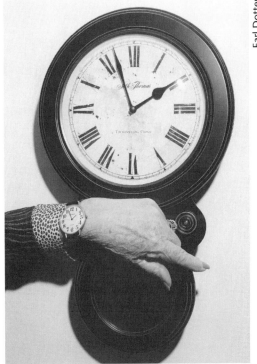

TELLING TIME

There are three basic options for telling time: large-print, tactile, or talking watches and clocks. There are many types of watches and clocks available to meet almost every need,

Time pieces with large numerals make telling time much easier.

and the watches are available in women's and men's styles. Some talking watches have alarms, calendars, or even the temperature. Atomic clocks that reset themselves when the time changes are also available. It may be possible to buy such devices from mainstream retailers such as department stores or discount stores. If not, check out the specialty catalogs listed in the Resources section.

Keep in mind, however, that the red displays of many of these devices are difficult or impossible for many people with low vision to read. Some people are better able to see green digital displays, so it is important to try them out and have your older relative make the best selection. Make sure that the clock your older relative buys is easy to set and reset—a task that sometimes can be complicated for anyone, regardless of eyesight!

Although the agency vision rehabilitation therapist may have provided instruction in how to use a timepiece, you may need to help your older relative practice telling time so that he or she feels more confident.

BRUSHING TEETH

You may not have thought of this before, but getting the toothpaste onto the toothbrush can be tricky when you have trouble seeing, and white, shiny bathroom fixtures can make it even more difficult. The following techniques make this everyday task a little easier:

- **Use a dark-colored or striped toothpaste to contrast with white toothbrush bristles, or vice versa.**
- **Hold the bristles of the brush between the thumb and forefinger while squeezing the toothpaste onto the brush.** An alternative is to squeeze the toothpaste onto a forefinger and then put it on the brush or to squeeze a small amount of toothpaste into the palm of the hand and then scoop up the toothpaste onto the bristles of the toothbrush.
- **If your older relative is the only one using the toothpaste, he or she may prefer to squeeze it directly into the mouth.**

HAIR CARE, MAKE UP, AND SHAVING

Knowing that they look their best can be important for the self-esteem of people who are coping with recent vision loss. These tips can help with everyday personal care:

- **Use a magnifying mirror to enlarge the face and head area.**
- **Drape a towel of contrasting color around the shoulders to make the head and hair more visible.** Alternatively, install a high towel bar across from the mirror in the bathroom and hang a contrasting towel on it to provide contrast when viewing the image in the mirror.
- **When applying makeup or shaving, use facial features such as the nose and chin as landmarks** to determine where to make the application or place the razor.
- **Use an electric razor for shaving for safety.**
- **Tactile markings or large-print labels can be used for identification of various grooming items** such as cosmetics and lotions.

DOING LAUNDRY

The easiest way to sort laundry is to immediately place white and dark clothing each in separate laundry bags when they are taken off and are ready for laundering. This eliminates sorting at washing time. Other suggestions and adaptations include the following:

Measuring Laundry Detergent

- **Use a measuring cup to measure dry and liquid laundry detergents.**
- **Measure over the washer so that any excess will still go into the wash.**
- **Try detergent tablets or pre-measured tablets with detergent.** Be aware that, depending on the brand, they may contain other laundry ingredients as well, such as fabric softener or stain fighters.

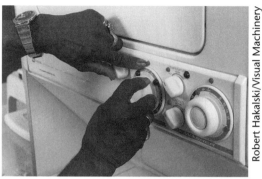

The most frequently used settings of washers and dryers can be marked with tactile dots.

Robert Hakalski/Visual Machinery

Marking and Setting Washer and Dryer Controls

- **Like the stove, washer and dryer settings can be marked tactilely.** You can use the product called Hi-Marks, which forms a raised mark when it dries. Your older relative will be able to feel when the dial points to the correct setting.
- **To make identification easier, mark only the most frequently used settings.**

GETTING AROUND INDOORS AND OUT

As described in Chapter 5, there is an entire specialty known as orientation and mobility (O&M) training dedicated to teaching people with visual impairments to know where they are in the environment and travel independently and safely. Even so, there are many things that you can do to help your older relative get used to moving around, either independently or with assistance, especially in familiar indoor environments such as his or her own home.

Individuals who have experienced vision loss can often become disoriented and be unsure of exactly where they are. Due to loss of depth perception or contrast sensitivity, they may find it difficult to detect the depth of curbs and steps, so they may encounter balance problems as well. Some techniques that can help them feel comfortable getting around may require orientation to the environment, the assistance of a sighted guide, the use of trailing and protective techniques, or some combination of techniques. As described in Chapter 5, advanced techniques such as training in the use of the long white cane is provided by an orientation and mobility specialist, and the use of dog guides is taught at special schools.

ORIENTATION TO THE ENVIRONMENT

You may need to orient your older relative to the environment—even in his or her own home at first—by helping him or her locate items in a room using the clock method or some other method that makes sense to him or her. Rooms that have color contrast between the walls and furniture may be easier for your older relative with low vision to navigate. (Chapter 7 talks more about making changes around the house that will help your older relative to move around more easily.) You may need to remind your older relative how many steps there are from the bathroom to the bedroom or living room. There may be landmarks, such as the back of a sofa, that you can use to help the person find his or her way around more easily.

TRAILING AND PROTECTIVE TECHNIQUES

Trailing is a technique that your older relative can use to feel safe and keep from bumping into anything when walking alone down a hallway, for example, from the bedroom to the bathroom. Have your older relative extend his or her arm about a foot in front and lightly touch the wall with the back of his or her hand. By trailing his or her hand along the wall while moving, he or she will avoid moving off course. You might also want to suggest using a tactile cue, such as a ribbon, on the handle of the bathroom door, to make it easier to find the door.

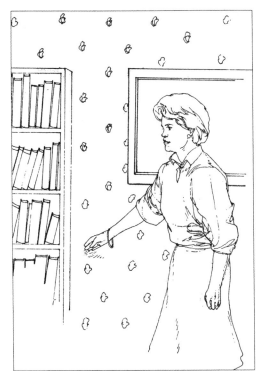

Trailing along a wall with the back of a hand allows an individual to keep from walking into objects in the middle of the room.

While trailing, your older relative can use a technique called the "upper protective" technique to protect the upper part of the body and face and help him or her feel safer. This technique is done by extending

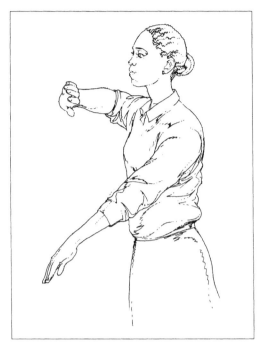

The upper and lower body protective techniques protect the head and lower body from injury while walking.

whichever arm is stronger straight ahead, bending it and bringing it toward the opposite shoulder, holding it about 8 to 10 inches away from the body with the palm turned outward. Then the arm is lifted so it is in front of the face, as high as the forehead. In this position the arm protects the head and upper body from injury should your relative bump into something, such as an open cabinet door, while walking. The fingers on the extended hand should be curled to avoid injury to the fingers, and the fingers and the entire body should be relaxed.

There is also a lower body protective technique. In this technique, the stronger arm is positioned at the navel and then extended out about 8 to 10 inches, with the palm facing the body. This technique will protect the lower body from injury. For maximum protection, your older relative can use both techniques together.

SIGHTED GUIDE

Sighted guide (sometimes called "human guide") is a technique you can use to guide your older relative in any unfamiliar environment or any time your older relative may need assistance getting around. You should let your older relative take your arm, just above the elbow. You will then be able to walk about a half step in front, so that you can guide and protect the older person.

When you are guiding your relative to a chair, describe the chair and its location and then put the older person's hand on the back. The visually impaired person should move the back of his or her hand across the seat to see that nothing is on it and it is safe to sit down. Your older relative can then seat him- or herself. If getting seated at a table, you as guide should place one of

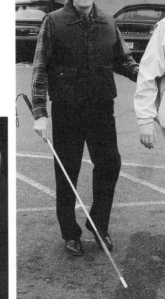

Earl Dotter

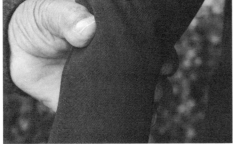

In the sighted guide technique, the person with vision loss grasps the guide's arm just above the elbow (left) and walks a half step behind (right).

the older person's hands on the back of the chair and one on the table edge.

When going through a narrow spot or doorway, tell your older relative that you are going through a narrow area and move the arm that your relative is grasping behind your back. This will guide your older relative to step directly behind you, and you can then move through the door in single file.

When getting into a vehicle, place one of the older person's hands on the door and one on the seat. You can also show your older relative the top of the car so he or she can judge how to avoid bumping his or her head. Explain which way you are facing and whether you are getting into the back or front seat.

One final piece of essential advice about guiding someone who is visually impaired: It can be very disconcerting and disorienting to a person who is visually impaired to suddenly find him- or herself alone in the middle of a room. Never leave a person with vision loss without telling him or her you are leaving.

THE LONG WHITE CANE

People who are experiencing vision loss are encouraged to use a long white cane to travel and for safety. Long white canes with red tips are universally recognized as being used by individuals with vision loss. When used properly, canes can also provide critical information about the environment by helping an individual detect obstacles, steps, or curbs. The efficient and safe use of the white cane in the outdoors is best learned from an O&M specialist, however, who can help with the proper selection of a cane and who is specially trained to teach these skills to individuals with vision loss. If your older relative needs to learn to use a long white cane to travel outside the home, or requires more than simple orientation to the indoor and immediate outdoor environment, contact a vision rehabilitation agency about an appointment with an O&M specialist.

Although canes can be ordered through catalogs, it is not to your older relative's advantage to order from a catalog without the assistance of an O&M specialist. The O&M specialist will make sure that your older relative obtains the proper cane for his or her height. In addition, your older relative may have other physical disabilities and may need to use an orthopedic cane as well. The O&M specialist can provide information on how to travel safely under these conditions. As with having eyeglasses or a magnifier prescribed and "fitted" by a low vision specialist rather than buying them off the shelf at a drugstore, it is better to have a cane selected by a professional.

DRIVING

For someone who has driven all of his or her life, having to give up driving—and the sense of independence that it entails—is probably one of the most difficult aspects of losing one's vision. There are no easy solutions. Your older relative can work with an O&M instructor to learn to use the local public transit system if there is one available. Also, most urban communities have a door-to-door paratransit system for medical appointments. You will need to work with your older relative to find out about eligibility requirements.

Senior programs often provide transportation for grocery shopping and for other activities, such as participating at a senior center or congregate dining program. You can call the Eldercare Locator number (800-677-1116) furnished by the Administration on Aging to find out more about transportation providers in the area where your older relative lives.

OPTICAL DEVICES

Optical devices utilize lenses that are stronger than prescription eyeglasses to help people with vision loss make the most of their remaining sight. Examples of optical devices are handheld or stand magnifiers to enlarge print or telescopes for seeing objects at a distance. Rather than attempting to buy any kind of optical device off the shelf, it is better to consult with a low vision specialist to determine what type of magnification, if any, would be useful for the types of tasks that your older relative wishes to undertake. For example, reading requires a different device than does viewing objects at a distance.

The low vision specialist can also provide essential training in how to use an optical device. A low vision therapist at a vision rehabilitation agency can provide follow-up instruction. Training and practice are required to learn how to use any adaptive device, so, although using an optical device can be tiring or frustrating at first, don't let your older relative give up before he or she has done both.

ADAPTIVE DEVICES

A number of nonoptical adaptive devices have already been mentioned in describing how to do everyday tasks. These are different kinds of nonoptical products that have been adapted to for easier use by people with impaired vision. One category of devices includes ordinary tools, devices, or other items that are labeled with larger than usual letters and numbers; some products may have tactile markings as well. Such large-print devices include
- large-print calendars
- easy-to-read weight scales with large, lit numbers
- large-print address books
- large-print rulers and tape measures
- easy-to-read blood pressure monitors

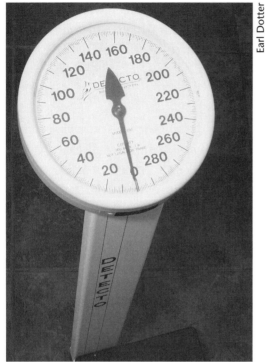

Earl Dotter

There are many products available with large print or large numerals, such as this easy-to-read weight scale.

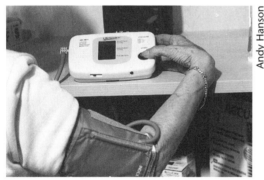

Andy Hanson

This blood pressure monitor is just one of many talking devices that are available for people with vision loss.

- low vision keyboards
- syringe magnifiers
- jumbo thermometers

Other so-called talking devices, which use synthetic speech to speak aloud measurements or text, help the older person carry out such diverse tasks as telling time, weighing oneself, taking temperature, measuring liquids, or checking blood sugar level. Examples of devices that talk include

- weight scales
- caller ID for telephones
- blood pressure and glucose monitors
- dictionaries
- digital thermometers
- voice label scanners that can describe products such as the contents of a can
- prescription bottles
- pedometers
- calculators

These devices can be ordered from the specialty catalogs listed in the Resources section at the back of this book.

In summary, your older relative can learn to do his or her everyday tasks independently using special or adapted skills, with limited assistance, or with the use of one or more of the adaptive devices mentioned in this chapter. Professionals such as vision rehabilitation therapists and O&M specialists will be able help your older relative find the best ways to accomplish what he or she wants to do, but following the suggestions in this chapter, there are many things that the two of you will be able to do on your own. In fact, some of the techniques and devices discussed in this chapter may prove to be the key to helping your older relative start over again. As the daughter of an older woman with diabetic retinopathy put it, "Just give me some suggestions and somewhere to go to find the resources."

In addition to these suggestions, take a look around your older relative's home and environment to see how it can be reorganized or adapted to support safe and independent functioning. This can make a tremendous difference in his or her ability to function independently. Suggestions about how to do this will be covered next.

Chapter 7

A Home that Supports Independence

Leon Felder recently lost his wife of 50 years to cancer. Not long afterwards, he had a stroke and lost a good deal of vision, and this has caused him to have some balance problems. Nora, his only daughter, wants him to move into a retirement home or assisted living facility near her.

"Nora, I just don't want to move," he explained. "I know I don't get around as well as I did before the stroke, and I don't see so well, but I'm sure I can stay at home."

"I don't know, Dad," she replied with concern. "I'm glad you're so optimistic, and I know you've had some training in cooking skills, but I worry about you. I wish I could continue bringing your meals over, but driving an hour back and forth every couple of days is becoming unmanageable. I wish you could move in with us, but now that Greg and Jason are both teenagers, there's not a square inch of extra room! I don't know what the alternatives are. I'm worried you're going to hurt yourself."

"I understand your concern. I'm concerned as well. That's why I want to tackle this head on. I was an engineer for 50 years, and I'm used to solving difficult problems. With the orientation and mobility training I've had, I've already figured out a way to mow the lawn safely. I'm ready to reorganize the house. I just need some help to set it all up."

"Okay, Dad. Let's give it a try. I'll come over this weekend and we'll arrange things to suit your needs—starting with the kitchen!"

"All right, Nora," he laughed. "Fair enough. Bring those two big boys of yours to help—if they can spare some time for their old grandfather!"

Like Nora, you may feel anxious about the safety and well being of your parent or other older relative if he or she lives alone. You may find yourself looking around your father's house or apartment and wondering how in the world it could ever be made safe. Trips and falls are a concern for all older people, and when someone is experiencing vision loss, ordinary household objects can become obstacles. Learning some techniques and strategies that will help to make your older relative's home safer and easier to navigate will help both of you feel more secure.

When Nora looks around her father's home, she sees hazards, but with the information in this chapter, you can look around and see solutions. Although vision loss does necessitate that some things around the house need to change, it does not mean that an older person must give up his or her independence. Your older relative's home can be organized and rearranged for maximum safety and independent living without spending a fortune. With a little common sense, you and your older relative can arrive at simple solutions that will help him or her stay safe at home, even when no one else is around.

Even if it is necessary for your older relative to move to a retirement community or assisted living facility, he or she will still need to carry out some daily tasks independently, and you can help within these residences as well. Moving to an unfamiliar environment in a new neighborhood is especially difficult for older people experiencing vision loss, and the techniques described in this chapter will be helpful in that environment as well. These suggestions may need to be introduced gradually, but throughout this entire process, remember that the one message you want to be sure to communicate clearly is: "I want to support you in your independence as best I can."[1]

BASIC SAFETY TIPS

Safety for your older relative is probably one of your biggest worries. Interviews with adult children of older parents with vision loss reveal that safety is their number one concern, with safety issues involving cooking and injuries due to falls topping the list. Ensuring that your older relative's environment is as accident proof as possible is critical, and this chapter will show you how to do it. Before you delve into of the details of home adaptation, however, read through the accompanying list of basic safety tips. They will help orient you to the whole process.

SAFETY TIPS FOR THE HOME

- **Remove small area rugs anywhere in the house or apartment.** They are a frequent cause of trips and falls.
- **Move furniture from the middle of a room to the wall to create an open pathway.** Eliminate obstacles or tripping hazards such as coffee tables in the middle of the living room or electrical cords stretched across pathways.
- **Use mats with nonskid surfaces in the tub or shower.** Also, make sure that the color of the mat contrasts with the color of the tub, so that it will be easier to see.
- **Consider installing additional lighting.** Adequate lighting is critical for people with usable vision, especially on stairways, in the kitchen, and in the bathroom.
- **Be aware of glare.** Eliminate glare caused by natural sunlight or lamps on shiny surfaces, such as glass table tops, highly polished floors, or the television screen.
- **Create color contrast among the things in the environment using color or patterns, for example, between wall coverings and furniture.** To heighten contrast between a white wall and a beige couch, for instance, use a contrasting dark-colored throw over the back of the couch or dark pillows.
- **Mark the edges of steps with a strip of contrasting paint.** Bright yellow and orange work best. You often see these strips on steps in public places, since steps are frequently the site of falls.

ADAPTING THE HOME ENVIRONMENT

At the end of this chapter you will find a Home Survey Checklist that you can use to determine how safe and functional your older relative's home is. Use the survey to identify areas that need improvement. Simple changes can mean the difference between an environment that's difficult to navigate and a safe, functional one. The suggested alterations won't cost a great deal of money, either, and you shouldn't need to refurnish your older relative's home or apartment. A few easy and relatively inexpensive changes can improve the environment immensely.

Conduct this survey with pen in hand and in the company of your older relative. That way, you can discover the specific trouble spots he or she has around the house and how they are related

---

SAFETY TIPS FOR THE HOME (*continued*)

- **Encourage your older relative to use a long white cane to locate potential hazards in the environment. Encourage the use of the self-protective techniques** described in Chapter 6 to prevent bumping into objects, especially around the head or face.
- **Remind yourself and others in the household to close doors and drawers completely,** to prevent the possibility of walking into them. Other doors throughout the home should be completely open or completely closed—but not left ajar.
- **Remove flammable or combustible items from around the cooking area in the kitchen.**
- **Practice operating a stove safely with your older relative.**
- **Install smoke alarms, carbon monoxide detectors, and fire extinguishers.** Make sure that your older relative knows where they are and how to use them.
- **Clearly label cleaning products, insect sprays, and other similar items with large print, or other labels for easy identification and store them together in one location.**
- **Mark the hot water setting in the tub with tactile or high-contrasting color identifications.** Check the hot water temperature to make sure it is set at a safe level.

to his or her particular type of vision loss. For example, glare affects people with cataracts in a different way than it might with other types of vision loss. Some people are extremely sensitive to light, while others need lots of light to see adequately.

There are eight key elements in the home environment that can be utilized and adjusted to enhance the functioning of people with vision loss,[2] which will be addressed in the remainder of this chapter:

- **lighting**
- **glare**
- **color contrast**
- **labels, lettering, and marking**
- **organization**
- **use of texture and touch**
- **environmental cues and techniques,** such as sound and smell
- **safety issues**

By applying strategies based on some or all of these eight principle elements (depending on your older relative's needs, as revealed by the Home Survey), you will create a home environment in which it is safer to navigate and easier for your older relative to find what he or she needs.

LIGHTING

Professionals who work with older people frequently find that older people use very little light; very often, practically speaking, they sit in the dark. People age 80 and older generally grew up with less light in their homes, and many are concerned about the high cost of electricity. Lack of adequate lighting might even cause them to think that their vision has deteriorated even more than it really has. By the time a person reaches 80, he or she needs 10 times more light than a younger person, as a result of the normal changes in the eye that were described in Chapter 2. Explain to your older relative that good lighting is extremely important, both for carrying out tasks more easily and increasing safety in the home. You and your older relative will see what a big difference it makes when you improve the lighting around the house. Formerly difficult activities will become easier, moving about will be safer, and it will be more comfortable for his or her eyes. Although well worth the extra cost, good lighting really doesn't have to be expensive, since the new natural light bulbs and compact fluorescent bulbs are longer lasting.

It is important to pay attention to two kinds of lighting. First, there must be sufficient overall lighting to move around safely. Second, it's important to have directed lighting for specific tasks, such as reading, using the stove, pouring a drink, or slicing an apple. Consider the following lighting recommendations:

- **Rooms should have more than one light source, so that lighting is dispersed throughout the room and there are no shadows or dark areas.**
- **Natural light (sunlight) is best for most tasks.** The closest approximation of natural lighting is now available from full-spectrum incandescent bulbs, such as Chromalux bulbs, available through specialty catalogs listed in the Resources section. The Reveal natural light bulbs produced by GE and Daylight bulbs by Sylvania are available in many grocery and hardware stores. These bulbs produce lighting that is similar to natural light and is whiter, cleaner, and good for all outdoor and indoor visual tasks.
- **Use incandescent lighting, such as the lightbulbs normally used in lamps, for reading or other close-up tasks such as sewing or playing cards.** This sort of highly concentrated light, which emphasizes the red/yellow/green end of the light spectrum, is best used in adjustable swing-arm and gooseneck lamps. Because it can create shadows and pinpoint glare spots, incandescent lighting is not recommended for overhead or general room lighting. High wattages may be needed to produce enough light to see clearly, however, and incandescent bulbs get hot.
- **Fluorescent light, which emphasizes the blue/violet portion of the light spectrum, is best for general room lighting.** It is mostly used in ceiling fixtures, although full-spectrum fluorescent bulbs are also available. Fluorescent lighting, which does not produce shadows, is cooler than incandescent light

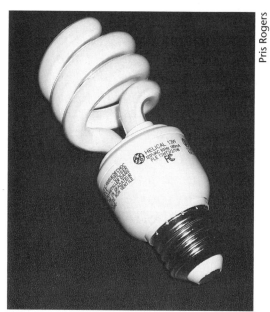

Pris Rogers

Compact fluorescent bulbs can be used in regular lamps and are good for reading.

and less expensive to operate. However, it cannot be dimmed as easily as incandescent lighting. Fluorescent lighting is not good for reading or closeup tasks and, unfortunately, it can flicker and produce an annoying strobe effect. However, newer compact fluorescent bulbs can be used in regular lamp sockets and are comparable to incandescent light for reading and produce much less heat.

- **Combination lights join incandescent and fluorescent lighting in one unit and are good for most everyday activities.** This combination creates a full-spectrum light and is the most comfortable type of artificial light.
- **Since halogen light is very hot and focused, and can cause fire or burns, it is not recommended for close-up tasks.** This whiter, brighter, and very concentrated light can be useful as track or recessed ceiling light, however.[3]
- **Use stronger lightbulbs or 3-way bulbs to provide increased lighting.** Make sure that the lamp is manufactured to use a high-wattage bulb, however, as many older lamps are not.
- **Place lamps in places where close work is done.** For example, use a flexible light, such as a gooseneck lamp, that can be positioned to focus directly on the task. Such lamps can be used in the kitchen as well as on the desk.
- **Install extra lights in the bedroom closet and other frequently used closets in other rooms.**

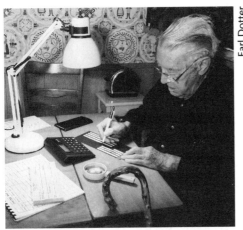
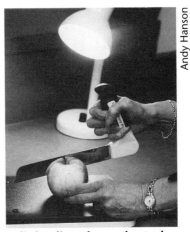

A gooseneck lamp can be positioned to focus light directly on the task, whether paying bills, reading a newspaper, or cutting an apple.

- Pay special attention to increased lighting over all stairways, where accidents are most likely to occur.
- Try to make sure the lighting level is consistent throughout the house to eliminate shadows and dangerous bright spots (which can interfere with vision).
- Install rheostats (dimmer switches) to allow light to be adjusted as needed.
- Be certain that light switches can be reached from the entrances to each room and from the bed to avoid fumbling around in the dark.

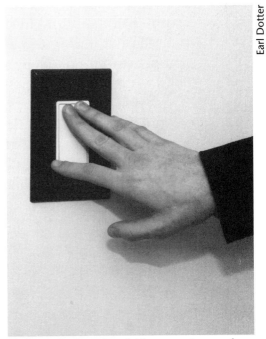

Light switches should be easy to reach from the door and the bed. They can be made more visible by using a contrasting color around the edges.

- Use a night light in the bedroom, hallway, bathroom, and kitchen, or anywhere else your older relative is likely to walk around at night.

GLARE

Minimizing glare will make your older relative's home much more comfortable. Glare is defined as reflected and uncontrolled environmental light that shines directly into the eyes and either causes physical discomfort or reduces visual clarity. Glare can interfere with eye comfort, physical safety, and the performance of many activities. It can be caused by any bright light hitting a shiny surface, such as a high-gloss tabletop, highly polished wooden floors, or the TV screen. You and your relative will want to survey the house for any glare and then figure out how to eliminate it. Reducing glare in the environment is critical, especially for people with cataracts or other conditions that can cause blurred or foggy vision. Here are a few suggestions for reducing glare:

- **Cover windows with shades, mini-blinds, or honeycomb blinds.** Mini-blinds are the best, since they can be adjusted during the course of the day to allow the proper amount of daylight into the room. Honeycomb blinds (an energy-efficient type of pleated shade) also work well if they can be moved up and down.
- **Reposition the television set so sunlight or lamplight is not shining directly on its surface.** This reduces the amount of glare from windows or other reflected light from a lamp.

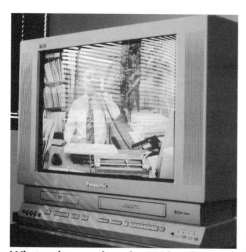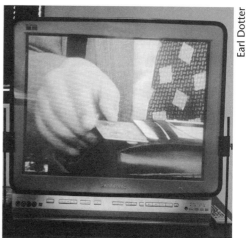

Earl Dotter

When glare makes the TV hard to see (left), simply turning it away from the light (right) can make a big difference.

- When going out, encourage your older relative to wear a brimmed hat or specialized sunglasses that reduce glare and cut the ultraviolet rays.
- Use a tablecloth on a table to reduce glare from tabletops.
- Encourage the use of nonglare wax on floors including hallways.

COLOR CONTRAST

Noticing a light-colored object, such as a white envelope, is always easier when it is sitting on a dark background, like a wooden desk, than when it is on a light-colored kitchen table—and vice versa. This is true for anyone, but especially for people experiencing age-related vision loss or other eye conditions. The use of color to create contrast was discussed in Chapter 6, and you will find that this principle can be applied in every room in the house to help your older relative get around better and locate items with more ease. Color can also provide important safety cues, in the same way that construction workers use bright orange or yellow tape or cones to serve as a barrier to a worksite. It can be used to indicate change in the type of floor surface, such as from wood to carpet or tile, or signal potential hazard, such as steps, by painting the edges a bright yellow or orange. Color can also be a factor in improving depth perception, which decreases with age.

When you and your older relative review his or her home using the Home Survey Checklist at the end of this chapter,

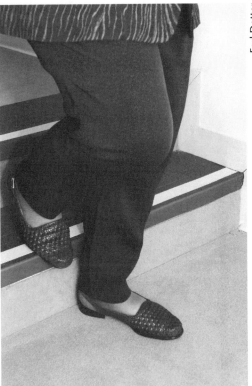

Earl Dotter

Color and contrast can be used to enhance safety in the home, for example, by placing a strip of a bright or contrasting color along the edge of steps to make them more visible.

you'll be able to determine where some changes in colors or patterns would help to create a residence that is safer, easier to navigate, and better suited for everyday tasks. Be sure to consult with your older relative before making any changes, however, especially in regard to something as personal as decor! Explain what you are trying to do, and ask for his or her suggestions. Here are some ideas to get you started:

- **Use dark bathroom towels as a contrast to white or lightly colored bathroom walls** to make it easier to find them.
- **Put light-colored objects against a dark background and vice versa.** For example, place a beige chair against a dark wood paneled wall, use a black switch plate on a white wall, or use black electrical tape around a beige switch plate.
- **Install doorknobs that contrast in color with the door.** If that isn't possible, hang a brightly colored ribbon on the doorknob so that it will stand out.
- **Avoid upholstery with patterns.** Stripes, plaids, and checks can be visually confusing. There's no need to

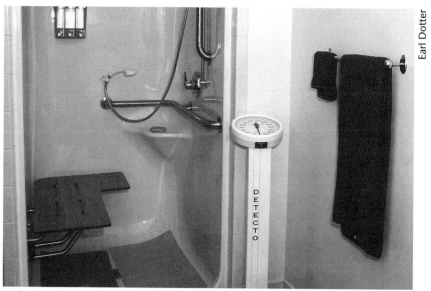

Earl Dotter

Color and contrast are important in the bathroom, where a dark towel will be easier to find against a light wall.

buy new furniture, however, if the color or pattern is not ideal. Draping a light towel over a dark chair, or placing a light colored pillow on the chair, can make it stand out from its surroundings so it can be located more easily.

- **Avoid patterned carpeting.** Patterns can be visually confusing to someone with vision loss. Also, locating a dropped object on a patterned rug can be next to impossible.
- **Paint thresholds with a highly contrasting color, and use color contrast on the edges of steps to make them easier to see.**
- **Make table settings more visible by using color contrast;** for example, placing a white plate on a dark tablecloth or placemat or vice versa.
- **Avoid using clear glasses with water or clear liquids.** Use a color-tinted glass or plastic cup, instead. Because water in a clear glass is difficult to see, it is easy to tip over while reaching out for it.
- **Use contrast in kitchen preparation areas.** Dark cutting boards work well on a light counter top. Cut dark meat on a white cutting board; hold up flour in a measuring cup against a dark cutting board or piece of paper to check the measurement.

LABELS AND MARKING

Distinguishing among objects that are similar, such as different varieties of soup cans in the cupboard, can be difficult with little or no vision. Identifying the right settings on the stove or the microwave can become a hindrance as well. Fortunately, these and a number of other difficulties can be solved through the simple process of labeling. There are a number of ways to identify and mark items around the house, some of which were identified in Chapter 6. Discuss these methods with your older relative to determine which ones he or she would like to use. You may have to use trial and error to see which methods work best, depending on your relative's type of vision loss and sense of touch.

- **Bold-line pens** can be used for labeling cans or to write instructions in large print.
- **3-D markers and Hi-Marks products produce raised and brightly colored markings** that can be sensed tactilely and can be used to mark items such as cans, thermostats, and settings on appliances such as stoves, washers and dryers, microwaves, and the like.
- **Raised dots can be used to mark objects or items such as medication bottles, remote controls for favorite channels, and the on-off switch for a television or radio.** These dots come on a peel off paper so they are easy to use.
- **There are also "talking labels," created with devices** that record information on magnetic cards. For example, the Voxcom records product identification information on a magnetic card that can then be attached to a pill bottle, clothing, or any item that your older relative needs to identify. To identify the item, your relative places the card in a magnetic card reader, and the information is read aloud by a synthetic voice. (These devices are available through the catalogs listed in the Resources section.)

ORGANIZATION

Many of us have at least one cluttered area in our home that we always plan to clean up. We often do not get around to cleaning as long as we are able to function by seeing or remembering where we put things or saw something last. However, a good organizational system is crucial for people with vision loss to find things around the house. You'll want to help your older relative keep things orderly and consistent. The best systems for organization are simple and easy to follow. You can assist your older relative with such organization tasks as rearranging a clothes closet or drawer to make it easier to identify clothing. As discussed in Chapter 6, it is critical in this process to communicate with your older relative and decide together how to reorganize things so that the system makes sense to him or her. Here are some tips for organizing various area of the home:

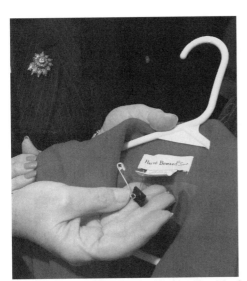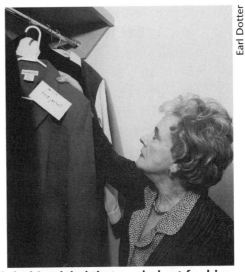

Earl Dotter

Your older relative can choose the kind of clothing label that works best for him or her, from different shaped tags (left) to hand-written index cards (right).

- **Use clothing tags to mark clothing.** These tags come in different colors and shapes, braille, and large print. (The catalogs listed in the Resources section contain a variety of types.) You can also use a 3"×5" index card to write, say, "red jacket" in bold letters and hang it around the hanger for identification. Or, you can pin the label on the sweater, remove it when wearing the sweater, and reattach the card after it has been worn or laundered.
- **Distinguish similar clothes with safety pins.** Suppose Leon Felder, the engineer mentioned at the beginning of this chapter, has three pairs of pants from the same manufacturer in three different colors, but now that he has vision loss they look identical. His daughter can set up a simple system to distinguish them from each other so that he can identify each one by himself. Leon can pin one safety pin to the label of the blue pair, two safety pins to the label of the brown pair, and leave the black pair unmarked.
- **Hang or place matching or coordinated clothes together as outfits.** Also, alternating light and dark clothing in the closet increases contrast and makes it easier to locate items.

- Use drawer organizers to put underwear, socks, and other items together. Egg cartons work well for small items such as jewelry.

- Establish a place to put essential small items, such as keys, remote controls, eyeglasses, and other frequently used small items. Put tape on the key your older relative uses most often, or color code that key in a contrasting color if he or she can see color. (Hardware stores often sell colored keys or colored rubber rings that can be placed around the heads of keys.)

- Organize the kitchen by using large-print or other types of labels for canned goods or frozen food. Group similar foods, such as canned fruits, vegetables, and soups, together in the cabinet.

- Arrange furniture in a way that makes it easy for your older relative to maneuver, and do not move it without checking with your older relative. He or she may have already positioned a chair as a landmark in the living room.

- Devise a filing system for bills and important papers that is easy to follow. For example, color code file folders or use large-print or braille labels. Dymo tape labelers, in braille or large print, are particularly useful. This device (available in specialty catalogs) has the alphabet on a wheel and can be used to spell out the words on self-stick plastic tape. The labels can then be placed on articles that your older relative needs.

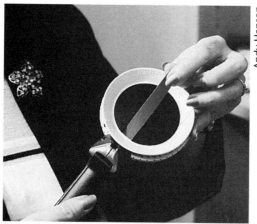

Andy Hanson

Dymo tape labelers, which come in braille versions, like this one, or large print, make self-stick labels in different colors.

- Keep track of appointments, important telephone numbers, and addresses in a systematic way. Several options are available, including large-print

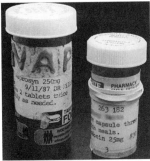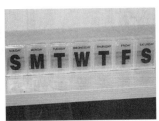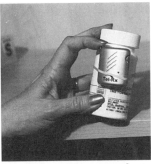

There are a number of systems your older relative can use to make sure that he or she can identify the correct medicine to take, including large print or rubber bands (left), pill organizers (center), and talking pill bottles (right).

calendars and address books. They can also be recorded on a small memo tape recorder.

- **Organize medication carefully.** You will probably be particularly concerned with managing your older relative's medication. A variety of pill organizers are available, some with alarm systems, to remind your older relative to take medications at a certain time. You and your older relative can also set up your own system to distinguish among a few medicine bottles. Different numbers or colors of rubber bands, for instance, can do the trick. Such systems can get complicated, however, when there are many medications to be managed. You can also write the name of the medication on a label on the bottle in large print, if your older relative remembers when the medication is to be taken. A newer option is talking pill bottles, which have become available over the last few years, that play a recorded message when placed in a special holder device.

USE OF TEXTURE AND TOUCH

It is a widespread myth that people who lose their vision automatically compensate by gaining more sensitivity in their ears, hands, or feet. It is possible, however, to teach oneself to become more aware of texture and ways to differentiate objects through touch and even smell. For example, your older relative may be able to identify his or her favorite clothing by touching the fabric or the buttons. People who have diabetes may have a harder time distinguishing between textures if they have neuropathy, or loss of sensitivity in their extremities.

As already noted, raised markings on stoves, microwaves, or thermostats can be used to give cues as to temperature settings and other settings. Also, your older relative may be able to distinguish various floor surfaces by feel and sound. These changes will let him know when he is passing from one room to another, for example, from the carpet of the living room to the tile of the bathroom or kitchen area.

OTHER ENVIRONMENTAL CUES

Your older relative may be able to use his or her sense of smell to locate things in the environment. Sometimes as we grow older, our sense of smell diminishes due to age-related changes in the olfactory nerves that control the sense of smell, so you will have to determine if this is a workable technique for your older relative. Smell is useful for detecting food that has spoiled; it is also helpful with safety issues, such as identifying the smell of a gas leak or of smoke. In additional, smell can be used to locate items or areas in the environment. The strong smell of aftershave lotion might signal that the bathroom is near, for example. Kitchen aromas are also good clues. When traveling outside, particular odors can signal that one is approaching a bakery or restaurant.

Using sound as an environmental cue is also very useful, unless your older relative is experiencing hearing loss. Sound can help your older relative pour liquids—the sound changes as the liquid rises higher in a container—or even differentiate between canned goods by listening as he or she shakes them. Sound can also be used quite effectively as a mobility technique to alert a person with vision loss to the approach of vehicles, for example. Talking devices with synthetic voices, such as talking scales, calculators, and clocks, are also available to help the older person cope with a number of everyday tasks, as discussed in Chapter 6. (You can find information about purchasing talking devices in the Resource section.)

Before she left, Nora and her father took a walk around his house together with the Home Survey Checklist. The next weekend, Nora came over with her sons Greg and Jason and a bagful of new products that she and Leon had agreed upon. As an engineer, Leon was delighted with the liquid level indicator, high-contrast kitchen tools, talking calculator, and the bright lamps. Greg and Jason enjoyed using the Hi-Marks and peel-off dots to mark the stove, microwave, and washer and dryer. They were able to improve visibility of furniture in the living room by placing a white towel on the back of Leon's favorite dark leather recliner and a red towel on what had been his wife's favorite light-green arm chair. Before Nora and her sons left, Leon agreed to consider letting them have a look at his clothes closets and drawers on their next visit.

HOME SURVEY CHECKLIST

Safe and comfortable living requires good planning, and the following checklist was designed to help you and your older relative design a safe and accessible environment. Conduct this survey with pen in hand together with your relative, so you can discover the trouble spots that are specific to his or her particular home and eye condition. Remember to always consult with him or her about any changes that you might want to make. Using your imagination and some of the suggestions in this and other chapters, most of the modifications can be done with minimal cost.

EXTERIOR

Entrance to Home or Apartment Building

_____ Are the curb and outside steps marked with a contrasting color?

_____ Do glass doors have markings on them to make them more visible?

_____ If there is a wheelchair ramp, does it have a nonskid surface?

Mailbox Area of Apartment Buildings

_____ Is the area brightly lit so residents can locate the right mailbox?

_____ Are the names and numbers large enough and easy to read?

_____ Are the boxes that belong to residents with vision loss identified with a brightly colored dot or a label?

Hallways of Apartment Buildings

_____ Is lighting uniform throughout the hallways? Is there glare in any area?

_____ Are doors or door frames a contrasting color to the wall? Are the baseboards a contrasting color to the walls?

_____ Are fire extinguishers located along one wall only and recessed so that an older person with vision loss can trail the opposite site of the hall without running into these obstacles?

_____ Is any equipment left lying around in the halls that can create a safety hazard, such as an unattended ladder or mop and pail?

_____ Are ramps identifiable by a tactile change in surface?

_____ Are exits clearly marked?

_____ Are floors cleaned or waxed with a nonglare, nonslippery finish?

_____ Are signs at eye level? Is there adequate color contrast and lighting to read them? Is the print large enough to be read?

Stairways and Elevators

_____ Are stairways clearly lit?

_____ Are the edges of steps marked in a contrasting color and texture to make them easily visible and detectable?

_____ Do handrails contrast with the wall and extend beyond the stairwell for extra safety?

_____ Are the tops of landings marked in a contrasting color and texture?

_____ Are the up and down light indicators of elevators easy to see?

_____ Can floor buttons in elevators be identified by both sight and touch? Are they in braille?

_____ Are floors also identified by an audible signal?

INTERIOR

General

_____ Are entrance thresholds flush to the floor? Have doorsills been eliminated?

_____ Are doors and door frames a contrasting color to the walls to make them easier to locate?

_____ Has color contrast been used effectively with walls, baseboards, woodwork, and floor coverings to help your older relative find his or her way around?

_____ Have window treatments, such as mini-blinds, been selected to help to control glare and maximize natural light?

Hallways

_____ Is lighting uniform throughout? Is there glare in any area?

_____ Are handrails in contrasting color to the walls?

Living Room and Bedroom Areas

_____ Is there adequate lighting for your older relative to read, write, or carry out other tasks? (Note: What you think is adequate may not be for your older relative. You need to verify this by trying out different tasks with your older relative. For example, reading generally requires higher wattage bulbs, full spectrum bulbs, or a combination of incandescent and fluorescent lighting).

_____ Is glare a problem? What about from mirrors? Flooring? Bright sunlight on glass table tops?

_____ Are there any throw rugs that should be removed?

_____ Is there furniture in the middle of floor that could be an obstacle or tripping hazard?

_____ Has a place been designated in each room in which to keep keys, TV remotes, and other small items that are easily misplaced?

_____ Is the TV located in a place where the older person can see it easily and away from glare? Is it close enough to see? If not, can it be placed on a movable cart or stand with wheels?

_____ Have closets and drawers been organized to facilitate locating matching clothing?

_____ Have raised or brightly colored markings been applied to thermostats for heating and cooling?

Kitchen

_____ Has color contrast been used effectively with walls, woodwork, floor coverings, cabinet surfaces, and pulls in the kitchen?

_____ Have brightly colored or raised markings been applied to the stove and other appliances such as microwaves to facilitate cooking?

_____ Is there a system in place for organizing the cupboards and refrigerator items, such as the use of tactile markings, large print lettering, or other means to identify cans, items in the refrigerator, or frozen food items?

_____ Has the kitchen been equipped with adaptive equipment such as large-print or raised-line measuring cups and large print measuring spoons, long oven mitts, liquid level indicators for pouring hot and cold liquids, tomato slicers, color contrasting cutting boards, kitchen timers with large numbers, talking or tactile thermometers?

_____ Have any flammable or combustible items around the cooking area in the kitchen been removed?

_____ Have smoke alarms, carbon monoxide detectors, and fire extinguishers been installed? Does your older relative know how to use them?

_____ Are toxic substances, such as cleaning products or insect sprays, clearly labeled and identifiable and placed together in one area?

Office Area

_____ Is there a filing system for bills and important papers that is easy to follow? For example, file folders can be color coded, or large print or braille labels can be made using Dymotape labelers.

_____ Is there a system to keep track of appointments, important telephone numbers, and addresses in a systematic way? Large-print calendars and address books are available, as are voice memo organizers and magnetic card readers.

_____ Does your older relative have a writing guide set with signature, letter-writing, check-writing, and envelope-writing guides, bold- or raised-line paper, and bold pens such as 20/20 pens?

_____ Is there a good light available for close work? Incandescent bulbs, full-spectrum bulbs, or natural sunlight provide the best light for reading. Swing lamps and gooseneck lamps provide directed light for tasks such as reading, telephoning, and sewing.

_____ Is the telephone accessible for your older relative? Does it have large numbers, or is it programmed to dial automatically? If your older relative is hearing impaired, is it equipped properly with an extra-loud ring and voice regulator or a light to indicate that it is ringing?

Bathroom

_____ Has color contrast been used effectively with walls, woodwork, floor coverings, cabinet surfaces in the bathroom? For example, the use of dark towels against a light wall can provide excellent contrast and can absorb some of the glare in a white bathroom. Similarly a dark, nonskid bathmat on a light floor can add contrast to light-colored walls and floor.

_____ Are bathroom fixture handles, door handles, and soap dishes or dispensers in contrasting colors?

_____ Has the hot water setting in the tub been marked so it can be identified by touch or through use of contrasting colors?

_____ Is there sufficient and appropriate lighting in the bathroom? For example, fluorescent lights reduce glare and also provide more even lighting in a general area. However, incandescent lights are better for close work such as applying makeup.

_____ Is there too much glare?

_____ Are there nonskid mats in the bathtub?

_____ Is the bathroom equipped with adaptive devices such as a talking scale, pill organizer, or magnifying mirror?

_____ Is the mirror easily accessible without having to lean over a sink, for example?

_____ Have pill bottles been organized and properly labeled?

_____ Is the floor covered with a nonglare, nonslip floor covering?

Laundry Room

_____ Have brightly colored or raised markings been applied to the washer and dryer to facilitate their use?

_____ Is there a system in place to sort or organize clothes such as dark and light clothing or to keep matching socks together?

_____ Is there a place to hang and sort clothing?

_____ Are large print or tactile measuring devices available to measure laundry detergent?

_____ Are detergents and bleaching agents clearly marked?

Dining Area

_____ Has the table setting been designed to maximize contrast the tablecloth or table mats, plates, cups among, and silverware?

_____ Have contrasting colors been used to differentiate the floor covering and tablecloth?

_____ Can glare from windows be controlled?

Chapter 8

Vision Loss and Other Health Conditions

Rose Chang is 75 years old and has age-related macular degeneration. She lives alone in a small apartment near her daughter Mei and her family. Mrs. Chang was having trouble adjusting the dials on the stove and finding small objects in her apartment. She couldn't read books, mail, or her own handwriting. In addition, visitors had to knock loudly several times before she answered the door, and the volume on the television was always very high. Once, when she had a small fire in her apartment, she did not hear the smoke detector. Luckily, her neighbor, who had a key to the apartment, smelled the smoke and alerted Mrs. Chang to the fire.

"I'm not going to the senior center any more," she told Mei when her daughter visited soon after. "It's too noisy there, and I can't hear what people are saying."

"But, Ma," protested Mei, "you've already stopped going to church. You don't want to visit me because you say you can't understand what Steve and the kids are saying. You can't just stay home all the time!"

"I can't understand the minister, so what's the point in going to church? It's embarrassing when people call out to me and I can't see or hear who it is. You're the only one I understand, and I can't make you repeat everything!"

That night, Mei called her brother and recounted the conversation.

"I'm so worried about Ma," Mei said. "She's becoming more and more isolated and depressed, and I don't think she's safe living alone. I think we'd better look into assisted living, or maybe a nursing home. I'm going to call the employee assistance program at work and see if they can recommend a place."

Instead of a nursing home, the employee assistance service told Mei about the local services for people who are blind in their home town. She arranged for a vision rehabilitation therapist and deaf-blind specialist from the Department for the Blind to assess her mother's independent living skills and determine what training and assistive devices might help her.

Two-thirds of older people who are experiencing vision loss also have another health problem, physical condition, or disability. The most frequently occurring conditions are arthritis, hearing impairment, high blood pressure, or a heart condition. Under any one of these circumstances, vision loss is one more compounding problem for older people and their families. If vision loss occurs after or concurrently with one of these conditions,

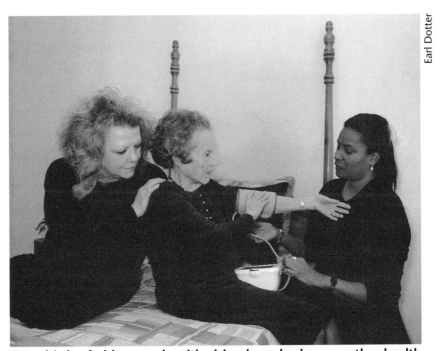

Earl Dotter

Two-thirds of older people with vision loss also have another health problem or condition, most frequently arthritis, hearing impairment, high blood pressure, or a heart condition.

your older relative may find it particularly discouraging. If an older person has a cognitive disability, such as Alzheimer's disease, a loss of vision can make the situation even more complicated. You can encourage your older relative to make the best use of his or her remaining vision and to seek vision rehabilitation services (see Chapter 5) while continuing to address his or her other conditions.

EFFECTIVE COMMUNICATION WITH HEARING LOSS

If your older relative has a hearing problem, you'll need to attend to this as soon as possible. As was discussed in Chapter 4, hearing loss can hinder communication between you and your older relative. Left unaddressed, it can affect your older relative's ability to adjust to his or her vision loss as well. Visiting a hearing specialist and obtaining a hearing aid or assistive listening device can make a world of difference in the ability to function on a daily basis.

People with severe hearing impairments often have difficulty following speech. Background noise, distance from the speaker, and poor acoustical situations contribute to their difficulties. Assistive listening devices can help by carrying the sound directly to the ear or hearing aid through a receiver. Assistive listening devices are specialized amplification systems that can improve audibility in specific listening situations. Generally they are best used for either interpersonal (one-to-one) conversations or communication in a large group. There are a wide variety of such devices; some are designed to be used with hearing aids and some are used alone. They are used in many situations such as meetings, classrooms, restaurants, parties, movies, tours, and religious services. (See the Resources section

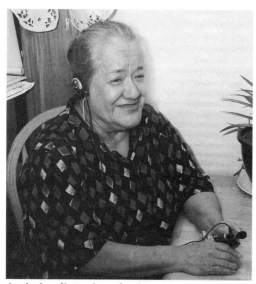

Earl Dotter

Assistive listening devices are amplification systems that carry sound directly to the ear or to a hearing aid through a receiver.

in the back of this book for a list of some organizations that provide information on hearing impairment.)

Some hearing problems cannot be helped by a hearing aid or assistive listening device, and you may need to seek help from a professional who can help your relative develop a way to communicate effectively. It is crucial for your older relative to see an audiologist to find out just what sort of hearing condition he or she has and what type of assistance is available. (Check the Resources section in the back of this handbook for information about where to find information and referrals assistance for hearing loss.)

Communicating with someone who has both a hearing and a vision loss can be difficult and frustrating. Try to be as patient and understanding as you possibly can. Remember, your older relative is having a hard time as well. It's important to figure out how you and others can communicate effectively with your older relative so that he or she will not become isolated. Indeed, isolation is one of the most difficult side effects of hearing loss. Discuss with your older relative what you can do to help him or her understand you when you talk. You may be able to present some options, such as seeking professional help.

Here are a few guidelines that will help effective communication with any older person who has a hearing impairment:

- **Speak slowly and very clearly.** Try not to slur your words or garble them. Enunciation is very important for a hearing-impaired person. Avoid talking while eating.
- **Avoid** speaking too loudly or shouting, which only distorts what can be heard. Speaking distinctly is the key.
- **Try using gestures and pointing as an additional way of getting your message across.** Of course, whether or not this is helpful will depend on the severity of the person's visual impairment.
- **Try to modulate your voice to avoid speaking in a high-pitched tone.** Hearing in the higher ranges disappears first when someone begins to lose hearing, so that deeper voices are easier to hear.
- **Never engage in conversation from another room.** You are likely to be misunderstood or not heard at all. Knowing that someone is speaking to you, but

not being able to understand what is being said, can be extremely frustrating and may even make your older relative feel that you don't understand or care enough to make allowances for his or her hearing loss.

- **Move away from background noise or competing discussions.** It may be hard for a person to hear in noisy situations where there is a lot of conversation and in rooms with poor acoustics. The use of a hearing aid does not mean a person hears "normally." Some devices magnify all sound, and background noise can effectively block out your communication.[1]
- **Minimize echo with environmental modifications such as carpeting or draperies.**
- **Allow for more "processing time" in the conversation.** Your older relative may need a little more time to assimilate what you are saying. When you're discussing something important, remember to make sure that your older relative understands what you are saying.
- **Be careful not to "talk down" to your older relative.** People often make the mistake of treating older people as if they were children or senile, especially if they have disabilities that affect their communication abilities. Remember, that having hearing and visual impairments does not affect a person's intelligence or cognitive abilities.

Mrs. Chang, the woman we met at the beginning of this chapter, was able to get the right combination of professional assistance with both her hearing and vision loss, and it changed the direction of her life:

While the vision rehabilitation therapist arranged for a low vision examination and helped Mrs. Chang with the skills and devices she needed to carry out daily activities, the specialist in deaf-blindness (both hearing and vision loss) arranged for her to have a hearing test by a certified audiologist. He prescribed hearing aids that dramatically improved her speech discrimination, and a special feature of the hearing aids (known as telecoils) allows her to make use of an assistive listening device in church, at the se-

nior center, and with the television and her Talking Book machine. She also acquired a loud ringing doorbell, a large-button phone with an amplifier, and a tone ringer control. When she takes her hearing aids out at night, a vibrator under her mattress will alert Mrs. Chang if the smoke alarm is activated. A separate vibrator under her pillow alerts her when the telephone or doorbell is ringing.

"I feel like I have been given my life back!" Mrs. Chang told her daughter.

ALZHEIMER'S DISEASE AND COGNITIVE DISABILITY

If your older relative has a cognitive disability, helping him or her cope with vision loss may be even more of a challenge. Building on current skills generally works better than trying to teach something new. For example, if your father has never used a microwave oven, it is unlikely that he will learn to use it at this point. Instead you may want to help him use a familiar appliance—such as a percolator for making coffee. He may need continual reminders—verbally or with a note in large print—about how much water and coffee to put in the coffee maker.

Here are a few suggestions that are generally helpful for people with cognitive disabilities or Alzheimer's disease:

- **Don't set your expectations too high.** Simple activities often are best, especially when they make use of the individual's current abilities.
- **Help the person get started on an activity.** Break the activity down into small steps and praise the person for each step he or she completes.
- **Watch for signs of agitation or frustration with an activity.** If someone with Alzheimer's disease gets upset, gently distract him or her to something else. Incorporate activities the person seems to enjoy into his or her daily routine, and try to do them at a similar time each day.
- **Eating can be a challenge.** Some people with Alzheimer's disease want to eat all the time, while others have to be encouraged to maintain a good diet. You may want to offer several small meals throughout the day in place of three larger ones.

- **Ensure a quiet, calm atmosphere for eating.** Limiting noise and other distractions may help the person focus on the meal.
- **Provide a limited number of choices of food, and serve small portions.**
- **Use straws or cups with lids to make drinking easier.**
- **Substitute finger foods if the person struggles with utensils.** Using a bowl instead of a plate also may help.

Vision loss and Alzheimer's disease can present similar difficulties. For example, Alzheimer's disease affects spatial perception. If your older relative is experiencing both vision loss and Alzheimer's disease, you might consider making some adjustments to his or her home, such as those in the following list and others discussed in Chapter 7.

- **Use color contrast between the wall and floor to help identify where one ends and the other begins.** Avoid monochromatic color schemes in which walls, counters, floor, and furniture are the same. When assisting someone with Alzheimer's disease, contrast is even more important than for people who only have vision loss.

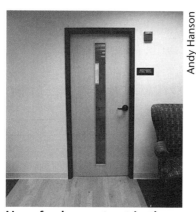

Use of color contrast in the environment, such as painting the trim of a door a contrasting color to make it more visible, is particularly important for people with both cognitive and vision losses.

- **Pay attention to light reflectance.** Using lighter colors (at least on the upper portion of the walls) can be extremely helpful in making the room lighter without adding glare.
- **Avoid distracting patterns in the wall and floor.** Try to go with a light or medium shade of flooring. Dark colors can be confusing in terms of depth and distance. (A dark floor will look much farther away than it really is.)
- **Consider landmarks that can serve as cues to help guide your older relative around the house.** For example, a sofa with which

your older relative is familiar and that will remain in the same place can indicate the path from the bedroom to the kitchen.

- **Call attention to doors you want your relative to use by painting the trim a contrasting color.** However, some doors may need to be made more inconspicuous, such as doors to areas storing dangerous or valuable items.

INDIVIDUALS WITH ORTHOPEDIC PROBLEMS

Older individuals who use walkers, wheelchairs, or support canes may require different techniques when learning the skills that will help them adjust to vision loss, especially when learning sighted guide (see Chapter 6) and mobility skills. You can help by learning sighted guide techniques that work with individuals with walkers, support canes, and wheelchairs. Here are some suggestions:

USING A WALKER

- **Talk to your older relative while guiding him or her.** Ask your older relative if he or she wants to walk independently while you describe the environment.
- **If your older relative is hesitant to use the walker independently, place your hand on one of the older person's hands and walk beside the walker as he or she moves.** Continue to describe the environment as you walk.
- **Walking in areas with glare may be difficult.** Ask your older relative if he or she needs additional assistance in these areas.

USING A SUPPORT CANE

- **When guiding your older relative who uses a cane for support, remember that he or she won't be able to grasp your arm with the hand that holds the cane.**

- **When guiding a person who is using a support cane, walk on the side away from the cane.** Your older relative may hold on to your forearm if he or she needs more support.
- **Continue to describe the environment as you walk.** If you are walking into the sun or in an area with a great deal of glare, the older person's vision

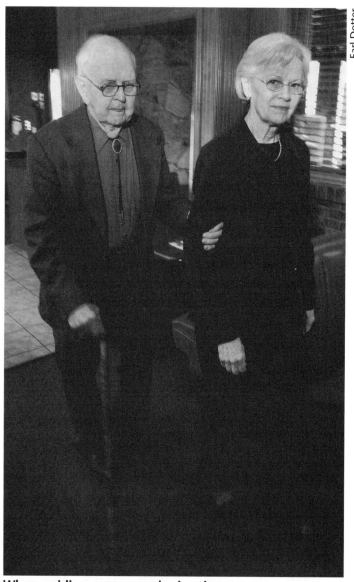

Earl Dotter

When guiding a person who is using a support cane, walk on the side away from the cane.

may be very blurred. Be prepared to assist by offering sighted guide.

USING A WHEELCHAIR

- **When guiding your older relative who is in a wheelchair, ask if he or she wants to be pushed.**
- **If your older relative wants to push himself or herself, you can provide guidance by putting your hand on one of his or her shoulders.**
- **Describe the environment as you walk.** Alert your older relative to obstacles.

GET THE HELP YOU NEED

You and your older relative will need to contact your local vision rehabilitation agency about setting up a rehabilitation program that meets your older relative's needs based on his or her specific combination of vision loss and other disabilities. Both the orientation and mobility specialist and the vision rehabilitation therapist will work with your older relative to devise an individualized plan of training. However, as discussed in Chapter 4, your older relative's desire to remain independent will have the greatest impact on this process. Be supportive, and remember that just because your older relative may have one or more physical disabilities does not mean that he or she cannot be successful in coping with vision loss.

In closing, consider the following true story:

Betty M., an 81-year-old music teacher in Orlando, Florida, needed extra income after retirement, so she started giving piano lessons in her home. Betty is hearing impaired, uses a wheelchair to get around because of hip and leg problems, and has recently dealt with the loss of vision in one eye and severe visual impairment in the other. With the help of the local vision rehabilitation agency, she has learned adaptive techniques to carry out routine tasks. Betty is still teaching piano, which not only helps her finances but also gives her satisfaction and a purpose in life.

Chapter 9

Support from Friends
and the Community

*I*rene Zhukov recently lost a great deal of vision due to diabetic retinopathy. Previously, she was very outgoing and enjoyed both going out with friends and having them over to play cribbage. Irene also enjoyed going to her church every week, and she was quite involved with her adult Sunday school class. Since losing her vision, however, she rarely goes out or entertains. Her daughter Ella is concerned about this situation.

"My friends don't know what it's like not to be able to see well," Irene told her daughter. "And, anyway, I don't want to be a burden on them. I can tell that my friend Alena, was embarrassed the other week when she had to read the menu to me. Plus, I knocked over two glasses of water by accident. Alena's pants were soaked. What if it had been scalding hot tea? I was mortified."

Since Ella was concerned that her mother was losing important social contact and support, she decided to call her mother's friend Alena to get her perspective.

"Your mother won't come out with us anymore," she told Ella. "We all miss Irene very much, but, to be honest, I'm a little relieved. I was so scared that your mother might trip and fall when we were out somewhere. Your mother's other friends and I wouldn't be able to lift her if she did. We don't even know how to help her out of the car properly. We have talked about this among ourselves and have decided that we just can't take *the risk. But I do try to call her every day to check on her. Sometimes she doesn't answer the phone, but I know she has to be there, sitting in that chair in the corner of her family room."*

Chances are that, although you love your family very much, no one understands you like your best friends. You probably share similar musical tastes, values, and basic assumptions with your friends, and this helps you feel at home in the world. This is no less true for your older relative who is experiencing vision loss. Older individuals who receive positive emotional support from both friends and family are more likely to adjust better to vision loss and to be happier. Family support is important, but without friends, older people are much more prone to experience loneliness. Loneliness is not only painful, but can lead to depression. Your older relative's friends are most likely upset, too, and missing their friend. Keeping old friends and making new ones is an especially important priority when someone is considering any change in living arrangements. One of the best things family members can do for their older relative is to help him or her stay connected to friends.

Unfortunately, when people experience vision loss, it can affect their friendships. Until they receive O&M training, it may be hard for them to get out, and not being able to drive can stop

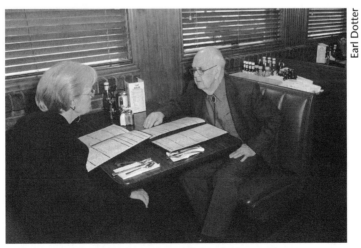

It is important to help your older relative stay connected to friends and maintain social activities.

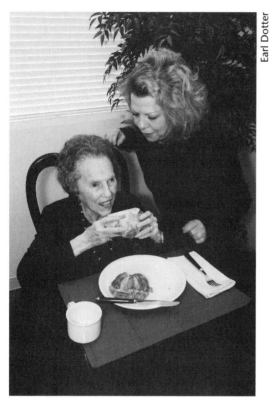

Earl Dotter

Mastering some simple eating techniques and possibly choosing an easy-to-handle meal can make your older relative feel more at ease and confident about eating in public.

them from participating in events at a senior center or visiting friends. Moreover, as noted earlier in this book, some older people feel embarrassed by their vision loss and consequently may avoid other people. Your older relative's friends might also feel uncomfortable around him or her since being with someone who is experiencing vision loss may remind them of their own vulnerability. They might truly want to be supportive, but not know how, or be afraid for your older relative's safety when they are together. Thus, for a variety of reasons, vision loss could cause both your older relative and his or her friends to withdraw from each other, eliminating critical sources of emotional and social support for everyone involved.

BECOMING COMFORTABLE OUT IN PUBLIC

What can Ella do to help her mother to retain her lifelong friends? First, Ella can make sure that her mother gets the help she needs to function as independently as possible. Once this happens, her friends may feel more comfortable about including her in their social activities. Have you ever noticed that when someone else is embarrassed or uncomfortable, you also tend to experience the same feelings? The same is true for friends of people who have recently lost vision. If Irene feels embarrassed or awkward, most likely her friends will, too. Helping your older relative feel comfortable living with vision loss is the first step to take toward maintaining his or her friends and social support. The rehabilitation training and skills discussed in the previous chapters will provide your older relative with a sense of independence, self-esteem, and general level of comfort that will put his or her friends at ease as well.

Many people who experience vision loss dread going out in public. They may feel conspicuous and vulnerable to pitying stares. There is also something about eating in public that makes many people feel particularly exposed. For people who have lost their vision, the fear of knocking over a glass, spilling something on themselves or someone else, or being unable to see what is on the plate can be intimidating and overwhelming. Mastering the simple eating techniques discussed in Chapter 6 will make your older relative feel more at ease

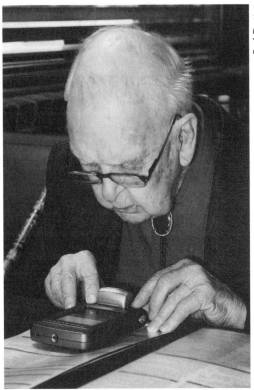

Some people are comfortable reading the menu with a lighted magnifier or portable video magnifier like this QuickLook.

and confident about eating in public; lunching with friends will be an option again. Also, ordering from the menu, when one cannot see, is a major stumbling block, particularly if the light is dim. Some people would rather choose an item that is typically served in most restaurants than have someone read the menu to them. Others are comfortable reading the menu with a lighted magnifier. Your older relative might want to plan ahead, choosing a menu item that is relatively easy to handle—for instance, a sandwich instead of spaghetti with meat sauce.

Here are some other pointers about eating comfortably in public:

- **Encourage your older relative to ask for a braille or large-print menu.** Alternatively, ask the waiter to read the menu. If your older relative feels uncomfortable doing that, you or another friend can offer to read it aloud.
- **Ask the waiter to address your older relative**

directly instead of talking about him or her to the other people present—a frequent occurrence in restaurants.

- **Tell your older relative what is on the plate and the table and where everything is.** You can use the clock method: for example, bread at 5 o'clock or beverage at 1 o'clock.
- **Tell your older relative when something new is placed on the table and where it is.** Your older relative won't necessarily know when his or her glass of wine has been brought or the salads arrive.
- **Practice eating techniques at home with your older relative before going out in public.** This will help him or her feel more at ease.
- **Avoid seating arrangements in a restaurant or other social setting in which there is a great deal of glare shining into your older relative's eyes.** When you arrive at your table in a restaurant, ask your older relative which seat would be best—usually a seat facing away from a window.

EDUCATING FRIENDS AND FAMILY

In addition to helping her mother become more comfortable venturing out in public, Ella can assist her in giving her friends a little information that will help them to feel more at ease around Irene and to know how they can help her if she requires assistance. The list of tips for family and friends found in Chapter 3 provides good basic information that will help sighted friends and family members know what to do when spending time with an older person who is visually impaired. In a situation similar to Irene's, you or your older relative could make a copy of this list for friends or family members to keep. You might also want to add your own ideas to the list, based on your older relative's preferences and pet peeves in various situations, along with suggestions about how to improve situations. It might be the waiters who always ignore your father and ask *you* what *he* would like to eat. Or your aunt might be most annoyed by restaurants that have only the light of a tiny candle for reading the menu. Irene told Ella that she was most frustrated when she asked for directions to the ladies' room, only to be told it was "over there." Another way to help everyone feel more at ease will be for you or your visually impaired relative to teach friends how to walk comfortably with him or her using the sighted guide technique described in Chapter 6.

Also talk to your older relative about his or her preferences with regard to broaching the topic of vision loss to friends. Irene might prefer that Ella present some information about vision loss to Alena and her other friends first, just to break the ice, or, once she feels more self-confident, she might decide that she is comfortable speaking to them herself. Don't make assumptions about what is best for your older relative; always consult with him or her. Helping your older relative preserve dignity and control over his or her own life is critical to maintaining the self-esteem and confidence that will allow him or her to feel more confident and comfortable with friends.

An important part of making it easier for your older relative to keep in contact with his or her circle of friends is helping him or her to realize that he or she still has something to offer as a friend. Losing one's sight does not mean that one cannot offer emotional support to others, especially to longtime friends, by listening to some of their problems or personal concerns. Being consulted as a friend will help your older relative maintain self-esteem and self-confidence. Unfortunately, this is often difficult for friends to understand. People think they are doing their visually impaired friend a favor by not bothering him or her with problems of their own. More often than not, however, the opposite is the case. Helping a friend will make your older relative realize that he or she is a valuable, contributing member of a social network.

COMMUNITY SUPPORT

Your older relative who is experiencing vision loss is likely to need a certain degree of support from services that are available in the community to continue to live independently. If your older relative finds it difficult to ask for that kind of help, your encouragement and assistance can help get him or her started. For example, if Irene needed transportation services to see the doctor or get to church, Ella might initially need to find the right telephone numbers to call, set up the first ride, and write the telephone numbers in large print on a list near the telephone or tape record them.

"It's really important to help my mom stay in control of her life. For example, we got a fax machine for mom so she can send us her bills and we can tell her what to pay and how much. Mother feels relieved and yet in charge."

–*Cheryl G., Atlanta*

Irene also needs help with grocery shopping. Rather than doing the grocery shopping herself, or going with her mother, Ella might be able to find a local service through a senior center that provides a companion for shopping. Not only will Irene be able to do her own shopping, but she will also become more familiar with the services of the senior center and feel more comfortable there. Senior centers sometimes provide other services as well, such as someone who can read your older relative's mail for him or her. Being able to choose assistance from services in the community, rather than being dependent on family members or friends, will probably help your older relative feel more independent. There are different ways to get the same job done, and it is up to the older person to choose from various options. You can help by making sure that he or she knows what the options are and that it is okay to make his or her own choice.

When offered the possibility of visiting a senior center, some older people with vision loss might at first say something like, "Why should I go to the senior center? I won't be able to do anything there." They may be feeling uncomfortable with the idea of getting help from a community service or anxious about meeting new people. You might ease the way by bringing along your older relative's version of a common game, such as large-print Scrabble, playing cards, or Bingo. (There is more information about such games and other leisure activities in Chapter 10.) This will help your older relative break the ice with other people there and be able to participate in activities immediately.

Older people who have begun to experience vision loss

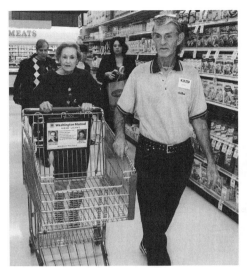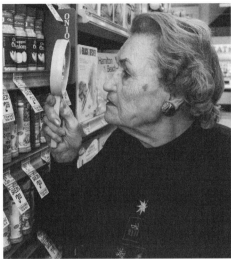

Being able to do his or her own shopping instead of depending on you will help your relative feel more independent. Some supermarkets provide assistance with shopping, and some senior centers can provide a companion to help your older relative.

have a new set of needs. They may find themselves in uncomfortable situations where it is hard for them to be clear about what those needs are and what assistance they are entitled to. They may suddenly have to deal with a number of community services, doctors, and individuals in social service agencies or cope with people who talk about them instead of addressing them directly. Speaking up for oneself is often one of the hardest things for anyone to do. Your older relative may find this especially difficult if his or her self-esteem is low at the moment and he or she is not yet comfortable handling day-to-day situations due to vision loss, such as having to ask whether a large-print menu is available in a restaurant. You can help by reminding older relative that it's okay to ask for help when he or she needs it. He or she can practice ways of communicating clearly and firmly, but politely; for example, "I am visually impaired and can't read the information you sent me. Could you please explain your service guidelines and tell me what time my appointment is?" Some vision rehabilitation programs may include discussion of such "self-advocacy" skills, in which people learn how to speak up for themselves in a direct and straightforward manner.

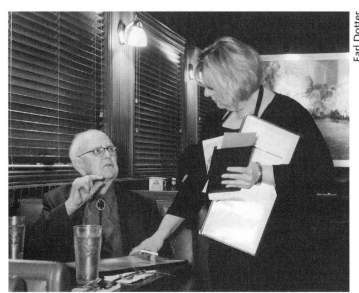

Earl Dotter

You can help your relative to feel comfortable about speaking up and asking for help, whether he or she needs a large-print menu or an appointment with a vision rehabilitation therapist.

INVOLVEMENT IN RELIGIOUS AND COMMUNITY ACTIVITIES

Many older people have enjoyed attending religious services all of their lives. Sometimes, however, they let vision loss stop them from going anymore. They may feel uncomfortable because they cannot read a prayer book, hymns, or other religious materials. They may feel anxious about not being able to recognize fellow worshipers. However, their vision problems need not stand in the way of attending worship services. More and more, religious organizations are providing materials in large print and on tape that can be ordered free of charge. In addition, assistive listening devices are also available in many places to help individuals with hearing impairments listen to the worship service. (See Chapter 8 and the Resources section for more information.)

Older people who can't drive themselves to a religious event might not feel comfortable asking for transportation assistance. But chances are, your older relative is not the only congregant who needs help, and there may already be a system in place to accommodate older people and those with disabilities. Many congregations have vans, and members often volunteer to transport people who are not able to get there on their own. Again, encourage your relative to ask for the help he or she needs. Helping your older relative stay connected with a church, synagogue, mosque, or other religious institution (as well as with other meaningful community activities and groups) can help sustain an existing source of support, maintain continuity during a time of difficult changes, and contribute to his or her self-esteem and sense of belonging.

Just as your older relative may feel uncomfortable with old friends or in a religious setting, he or she may feel ill at ease continuing involvement in clubs or associations—say, a political group, poker night, gym, or a reading group. Chapter 10 will talk more about how he or she can continue in these activities, while you may need to help by finding out what about the situation is particularly distressing and address these concerns. Encouraging your older relative to share some of the tips for family and friends (see Chapter 3) may help other club members to feel more comfortable. It might also help to point out to your older relative that others in the group may also be experiencing vision problems now, or will be in the future, or may have other health problems or disabilities. Your relative might end up serving as a positive example to others of how to cope in similar situations!

In summary, helping your older relative to maintain friendships and involvement in social activities is critical to the adjustment process—and to leading a satisfying life. But be careful not to push your older relative faster than he or she is willing to go. Sometimes, addressing each situation as it comes up is better than dealing with all of them at one time. As one daughter put it, "Mom has adjusted well, but she says she's 'a work in progress' and has to have time to sort through how to deal with issues as they arise, with the help of family and friends."

YOUR SUPPORT SYSTEM

Just as your older relative needs a support system, you need one, too. Providing emotional and physical support to an older relative, while often rewarding, can also be quite draining. Your spouse, your children, children, and siblings, if you have them, can provide you with a great deal of support. Sometimes, however, you may begin to feel that everyone needs more of your time until you are performing a juggling act! If possible, try to get your children involved in visiting your older relative and enjoying that time together. Even something as simple as involving your children in rearranging the living room furniture to accommodate their grandmother's vision loss can be enjoyable. Not only will they have a good time, but your children will learn to appreciate how important it is help others. And, if they're involved, they're likely to be more cooperative and understanding about why you need to spend some of your time away from home helping Grandma.

Don't forget that you are likely to need support from outside your family as well. You may feel that you ought to limit your own social life, but try not to. Sharing your feelings with close friends can help to reenergize you when you're drained.

Others who are struggling with the same set of issues can be a great source of support as well. Ask the agency where your older relative is receiving vision rehabilitation training if there is a support group for family members. If there is, drop in and talk to other families who are facing similar challenges. If one does not exist at your agency, consider asking them to start one. If you have the time and energy, offer to help in starting a group yourself. Chances are, there are many other people right in your area who could benefit. If the agency is not able to start a group because of limited resources, ask them if you may contact other family members to see if they would be interested in participating in such a group privately. (The agency might not be able to release names to you because of a confidentiality policy, but they may be willing to contact them on your behalf.)

Though the structure of support groups can vary from location to location, they should always provide you with two things: mutual support and information. Some sessions can be devoted to discussing feelings and experiences, while others can be more educational. Consider inviting professional speakers to meetings to talk about various age-related vision loss issues. They can help you comprehend some of the more esoteric concepts surrounding vision loss, as well as help you better understand the psychological aspects of what your older relatives are experiencing. (Consult the Resources section of this book for information about starting a group, such as the Hadley School's course on support groups.)

If you cannot find or form a support group specifically related to age-related vision loss, try to find a general support group for adult children of older people with disabilities or health problems. An agency serving elders in your community might maintain such a group. Even if most of the other people in the group do not have older relatives with vision loss, you'll likely find that you still have a great deal in common with the other participants. Anyone faced with the challenge of supporting an older person with a disability needs emotional support.

Most important, keep in mind that you need to take time for yourself. Treat yourself well, and make sure you schedule time to relax and enjoy yourself. You won't be able to support your older relative if you're burned out, stressed, and exhausted most of the time.

In summary, recognize that both you and your older relative need support throughout the process of adjusting to vision loss. Because vision is involved in almost every one of our daily activities, dealing with vision loss takes time, patience, and support from professionals, friends, and families. The good news is, the help is out there.

So far, this handbook has presented you with a number of tips that will help your older relative make adaptations to his or her life and home. But what about enjoyment? Being able to have a good time makes life worth living, and continuing to engage in pleasurable activities is one important way that we adapt to problems and losses in our lives. In Chapter 10 you will find out about how to help your older relative continue with valuable leisure activities.

Chapter 10

Enjoying Leisure Activities

Evita Garcia enjoyed few activities more than retiring to the backyard to read each day after finishing her housework. She spent blissful hours devouring novels in both English and Spanish. "The only thing I love more than reading is my children," she once told her daughter, Carmela. Vision loss changed everything.

Evita had lost all vision in one eye and had severe tunnel vision in the other as a result of glaucoma. More than anything, she was concerned about being able to continue reading. Carmela remembered that years ago, after visiting an aunt of Evita's who had gradually become blind, her mother had remarked, "I have endured many losses, but I couldn't handle losing my sight. Without my books, I would be lost."

Carmela watched her mother give up on reading after she was diagnosed with glaucoma and saw her fall into a listless depression. After a visit to her ophthalmologist, Evita was told that nothing more could be done for her vision. She began to feel even more hopeless, and Carmela knew she had to do something about it. "There must be a solution," she thought.

Leisure pursuits enhance everyone's life—young and old. They are an important part of our lives. In fact, having fun is necessary; we can't work and take on difficult challenges without getting a break now and then. This is especially true for your older relative who is experiencing vision loss, who simply needs to relax from time to time while he or she develops adaptive life skills in vision rehabilitation training. Keeping active is critical for a healthy lifestyle, and your older relative should be encouraged to remain so. There's no reason why, with a few new skills or specialized equipment, your older relative can't enjoy most of the leisure activities he or she always has, or even new pastimes.

Unfortunately, what happened to Evita in the example at the beginning of this chapter happens to many older people who are experiencing vision loss. Eye care professionals often say, "There is nothing that can be done"—when what they really mean is that nothing further can be done *medically*. Many people react by giving up on learning how to adjust to life with vision loss, assuming that they don't have any other options. As you will realize, having read this far, that is rarely the case.

Just as your older relative can learn to manage most daily activities independently, he or she can continue to enjoy leisure time. Losing vision does not mean losing physical or mental energy. Encourage your older relative to maintain his or her interests after the onset of vision loss and to cultivate new ones. Reading is just one example. Other activities include walking, watching television, doing needlework and sewing, playing board games or cards, gardening, attending social and cultural events such as the theater and concerts, and even participating in sports. The possibilities are endless.

Through the wide variety of services, special products, and alternative approaches that are available, leisure activities of all sorts are still possible. Hobbies, volunteer work, and membership in senior centers and in clubs and support groups are all viable options. There are even national organizations for people experiencing vision loss that focus on adapted sports—that is, sports that utilize special forms of equipment or rules—such as golf, bowling, and skiing. Although this chapter will present some of the possible options for leisure activities, there are many other sources of valuable information available to your older relative. Consult the Resources section at the end of this book for more information about organizations, products, and services.

THE ENDLESS VARIETY OF LEISURE ACTIVITIES

At first, your older relative might be apprehensive about enjoying leisure activities independently. Participating in an activity with your older relative that you both enjoy can get the ball rolling. For example, the two of you can dine out, attend a food fair, or see a show. Get some physical exercise by golfing, bowling, swimming, lifting weights, or going outdoors to walk in the park, fish, or ski. There is nothing to stop you and your older relative from listening to the radio, doing a crossword puzzle together, going to a poetry reading, attending a lecture series, or enjoying a football game. (Many people with vision loss listen to the play-by-play commentary on the radio about a game right in the stands of the stadium.) Attend religious services or take an exercise class together. Volunteer at a local charitable organization, go to a political rally, or get a manicure together. The possibilities are nearly limitless. If you haven't engaged in these activities together in the past, just make a suggestion to try one and see what happens. The following sections offer information about how to adapt specific activities for someone with vision loss.

READING

Reading is still very much an option for Evita Garcia. Given her extensive vision loss, the best alternative for her may be using Talking Books. Part of the National Library of Congress, this national program provides books recorded on cassette for people with vision loss or who are physically disabled and cannot turn the pages of a book. The books and cassette machine to play the Talking Books are provided free of charge by the National Library Service for the Blind and Physically Handicapped. Your older relative will need a special cassette machine, since these tapes cannot be played on just any tape player. Obtaining the machine and books, however, is a simple process.

To access the books and magazines provided by the program, a brief application is required. A physician, local librarian, or vision rehabilitation professional must sign the application. Your older relative can get one from his or her vision rehabilitation therapist, from the library, online, or by calling an 800 number.

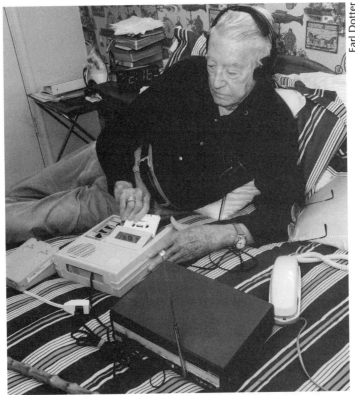

Earl Dotter

One reading alternative is listening to Talking Books on cassette, which are provided free of charge, along with the machine to play them.

(Contact information can be found in the Resources section.) Signing someone up for Talking Books is usually one of the first things the vision rehabilitation therapist does. Most people miss reading a great deal but do not know there is an alternative to printed books. The National Library Service also maintains a system of libraries that carry audio as well as braille books. Information about these libraries is available at the National Library Service Web site (www.loc.gov/nls) or through the *AFB Directory of Services for Blind or Visually Impaired Persons in the United States or Canada,* which can be purchased from the American Foundation for the Blind (see the Resources section) or accessed online at www.afb.org.

The National Library Service is in the process of developing a new digital format for its Talking Books, which is planned to begin distribution in the next few years. Digital Talking Books will have exciting features for listeners, such as the ability to jump forward or back by chapter, set bookmarks, and vary the speed of the reader's voice without affecting its pitch.

Many books are also available commercially on tape or CD at most bookstores. These do not require a special player, as the Talking Book program does, and cost about the same as a print book.

Large-print books are a good alternative for those who can read print in 16- or 18-point type. Most libraries now have a large-print section of the library. *Reader's Digest* and *Newsweek* publish large-print versions as well. Some publishing companies such as Doubleday Book Club have large-print membership divisions. The *New York Times* publishes an abbreviated weekly addition in 16-point type, available by subscription, which includes news highlights from the week. You may want to make note of the "Tips for Print Readability" when your older relative is selecting reading matter— or when you are writing something for him or her to read.

Using low vision reading devices is another alternative for individuals with low vision. Good task lighting is critical for reading, as covered in Chapter 7. Handheld or stand magnifiers are an excellent choice for individuals who want to read their bills or correspondence as well as their leisure reading. Although magnifiers and other low vision devices are available through catalogs and over the counter, it is generally advisable for a low vision specialist to conduct an examination for anyone with significant vision loss and to prescribe a device selected specifically for an individual's needs. The specialist can determine precisely how much magnification your older relative needs and provide training and follow-up in use of the device. Using a magnifier may seem simple, but it must be held at a precise distance from the printed material for the words to come into focus. Therefore, training in how to use a magnifier or other low vision device is critical. Without it, some people become discouraged, put the magnifier in a drawer, and give up on reading entirely.

Another alternative is a closed-circuit television system (CCTV), a device that uses a camera to magnify printed material. The printed material is placed on a flat tray, and a camera projects an enlarged image of the material onto a monitor, similar to a television screen. There are many different CCTV models available on the market today, including some that connect to a regular television set or computer screen. There are also portable versions that can be taken to the supermarket to read food labels or a restaurant

TIPS FOR PRINT READABILITY

Reading print can present specific challenges for your older relative with vision loss, depending on his or her specific eye condition. For instance, reading can be difficult because of a reduced amount of light entering the eye, a blurred image on the retina, or a defective macula (the central portion of the retina). Reduced light and blurring affects the contrast of the print against its background. Damage to the central retina interferes with the ability to see small print and to make the eye movements necessary for reading. The following are guidelines for making print more legible for individuals with these vision problems—as well as for people with good vision.

Print Size

Large-print type should be used, preferably print in 18 point, but at least in 16 point. Scaleable fonts on the computer make this easy to do if you are writing something for your older relative to read.

Font Type and Style

The goal in font selection is to use easily recognizable characters, either standard roman or sans serif fonts (without extra tips at the end of letters), such as Arial.

- Avoid decorative fonts.
- Use bold type, since the thickness of the letters makes the print more legible.
- Avoid using italics or all capital letters. Both these forms of print make it more difficult to differentiate among letters.

Color

The use of different-colored letters for headings and emphasis is difficult to read for many people with vision problems. When color is used, dark blues and greens are most effective.

Contrast

Contrast is one of the most critical factors in enhancing visual functioning, for printed materials as well as in environmental design. Text should

(continued on next page)

TIPS FOR PRINT READABILITY (*continued*)

be printed with the best possible contrast. Some older people are able to see white or light yellow lettering on a dark background. Others prefer black lettering on a white or ivory background.

Paper Quality

Avoid using glossy-finish paper such as that typically seen in magazines. Glossy pages create excess glare, which increases reading difficulty for people who have vision problems.

Leading (Space Between Lines of Text)

Double space between lines of text. Many people who are visually impaired have difficulty finding the beginning of the next line when single spacing is used.

Tracking (Spacing Between Letters)

Text with letters very close together makes reading difficult for many people who are visually impaired, particularly for those who have central visual field defects, such as people with age-related macular degeneration. Spacing between letters should be wide, such as that in mono-spaced fonts (fonts that have an equal amount of space allocated for each letter) such as `Courier`.

Margins

Many low vision devices, such as stand magnifiers and closed-circuit television systems, are easiest to use on a flat surface. When material is bound or placed in a binder, an extra-wide margin in the center makes it easier to hold the material flat for use with these devices. A minimum of 1 inch should be used; 1½ inches is preferable.

Research is still under way to determine ways of making text more legible for individuals with limited vision.

to read menus. Encourage your older relative to ask a low vision specialist or professional at a vision rehabilitation agency about the variety of choices. The prices vary widely depending on features, the range of magnification, and the size of the screen. The versions that use TVs generally cost less than $1,000. Stand-alone products generally begin in price range from approximately $1,800 for the black-and-white version; color CCTVs are more expensive. Many libraries now have CCTVs as well.

Electronic publishing, or e-publishing, is a new way to read books that people with vision loss can take advantage of. These e-books exist in electronic or digital files that can be downloaded into special e-book readers, personal digital assistants (PDAs), or even cell phones. Although the small screens of these devices can be difficult to see for people with vision loss, there are also special e-book readers and PDAs that allow people with vision loss to listen to e-books using speech output. Some e-books can also be read on computers using magnified text or speech output. Digital Talking Books, which allow the user to customize the font size of the text or play it in audio, are an alternative designed specifically for people with vision loss. These specialized e-books require a special device or computer software to play them, but in the next few years such players will become much more common, and, as already mentioned, these books are likely to replace Talking Books on cassette as standard reading

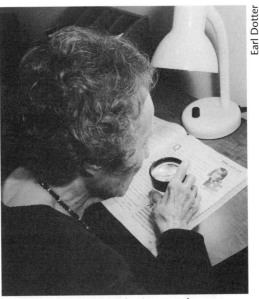

Earl Dotter

Low vision reading devices such as magnifiers are a good alternative, but they will be most useful if your relative obtains training in the use of a device that is prescribed for his or her specific needs by a low vision specialist.

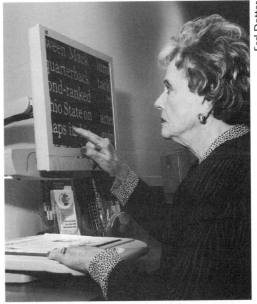

Earl Dotter

There are many types of CCTVs, which magnify the image of printed materials and display it on a monitor.

material for people with vision loss. The National Library Service (see the Resources section) has a fact sheet listing many sources of e-books, which appears on its Web site (www.loc.gov/nls).

MUSIC

Music is an activity that people can continue to enjoy both as a listening and a creative activity. For those who want to continue to listen to music, you may want to help mark a tape or CD player so that your older relative can operate it easily, following some of the recommendations for labeling and marking devices in Chapter 6.

For those interested in singing or playing music, the Library of Congress has a special music collection for blind persons as part of its free National Library Service of braille and recorded books and magazines. Music services include a circulating collection of braille, large-print, and recorded instructional materials and a subscription program of magazines produced in braille, on cassette, and in large print. (Musical recordings intended solely for listening are not part of the music collection, as these materials are readily available from stores and local public libraries.) For more information about the NLS Music Section see the Resources section of this book or the Web site www.loc.gov/nls/reference/factsheets/music.html.

RADIO READING AND NEWSLINE SERVICES

Radio reading services for people with vision loss are available in many areas of the country. Individuals who subscribe to these services have special radio receivers and can listen to daily newspapers and local periodicals read by local volunteers. These radio reading services often offer other types of programming of interest to persons with vision loss as well. (See the Resources section for more information.)

The National Federation of the Blind has established the NFB-NEWSLINE news service (see the Resources section), which is accessible by simply dialing a toll-free number. Dozens of newspapers—read by synthetic speech—are now available through this service 24 hours per day, 7 days per week. Individuals who are visually impaired are eligible for this free service by filling out a simple application.

WATCHING TELEVISION

If your older relative has some usable vision, he or she may still be able to watch television. Simply moving the screen closer and positioning it to avoid glare from the sun or from a lamp can make a big difference. Placing the TV on a rolling cart makes it easier to move. TV screen enlargers—special screens placed over a regular TV set to enlarge the picture somewhat—can be found in independent living catalogs. Another item that makes watching TV easier is a universal remote control panel, which comes with large buttons and has speech and voice-recognition capabilities. These make it easier to learn and memorize the positions of the settings on the remote. (See the Resources section for a list of independent living catalogs.)

VIDEO DESCRIPTION

Some television programs and films on videotape are available in versions that have a description of what a viewer would see on the screen inserted on the sound track. This narration, known as video description, is accomplished without interfering with the sounds and dialogue that are part of the program. Video description can make programs more enjoyable for individuals who are unable to see the screen, especially when there is a great deal of unspoken action. For some television programs, these descriptions can be heard on a separate audio channel—called Secondary Audio Program or SAP—that is available on most stereo television sets sold in the United States. Video described programs are also available on many public broadcasting and cable stations, and video described movies can be purchased or borrowed from some libraries and video stores. Some sources of video description are listed in the Resources section.

NEEDLEWORK AND SEWING

If your older relative enjoys needlework and sewing, he or she can benefit from specialized sewing techniques, magnification, and various special devices. Self-threading needles, different types of needle threaders (including some for sewing machines), and tactile or talking measuring devices can all help. A substance called Liquid Stitch is also available for repairing hems without sewing. All of these products can be found in catalogs and even in conventional sewing stores.

Making a few simple adjustments may mean not having to give up a valued leisure activity. People with some usable vision can benefit from the use of contrast by sewing with contrasting fabric colors or using a contrasting background for knitting or other crafts. CCTVs can also be utilized to see close, detailed work. Marking fabrics with Hi-Marks or using textured fabrics can also help. Have your older relative experiment to find out what works for him or her.

ADAPTIVE GAMES

Many games—including cards, Bingo, checkers, dominos, Scrabble, chess, and even Monopoly—are available in formats specifically designed for people with visual impairments. Large-print and tactile markings, including some in braille, are utilized to make these games playable. You can play these games

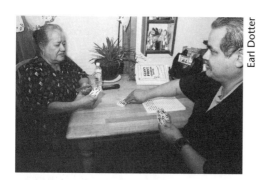
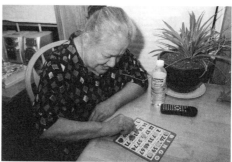
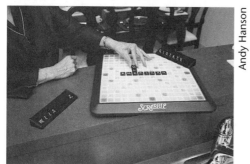
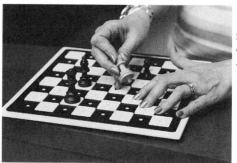

Earl Dotter

Andy Hanson

Many games are available in formats specifically designed for people with visual impairments, including large-print playing cards, Bingo, and Scrabble and chess sets in which the pieces are harder to knock over accidentally.

with your older relative using the adaptations and special devices as well.

GARDENING

Many older people enjoy gardening but may not feel up to doing it in a large open area. Growing house plants can be good alternative. Container gardening, a good method to use for growing vegetables or flowers in small spaces such as patios or porches, is also an option. Small salad greens are ideal. Cherry tomatoes and other fruiting vegetables, including peppers or eggplant, can be easily grown in containers, as can root vegetables such as baby carrots, radishes or spring onions. Flowers such as marigolds, zinnias, and impatiens also flourish in planter boxes, wooden barrels, window boxes, hanging baskets, or large flowerpots. Containers can be painted in high-contrast colors to help with identification. (Check out www.gardenguides.com/TipsandTechniques/container.htm for more container gardening tips.) The Hadley School for the Blind (listed in the Resources section) has correspondence courses on recreational activities including gardening as well.

Your older relative might also enjoy growing herbs, which can be identified through scent. Help him or her label plants with large-print markers or tactile indicators. Painting the tines of hoes or rakes white will help by providing contrast with the dark dirt. Your older relative might also need to wear a hat or sunshade to reduce the glare while gardening.[1]

COOKING

For many older people cooking may have been an enjoyable hobby in addition to a necessity. Preparing meals can still be a satisfying way to spend leisure time, once your older relative has received vision rehabilitation training and has learned about alternative techniques for food preparation.

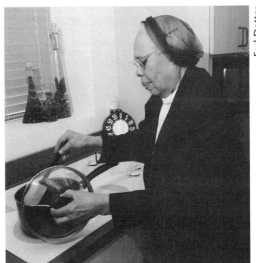

Earl Dotter

Cooking can be a satisfying hobby as well as a necessity.

SOCIAL AND CULTURAL ACTIVITIES

Older people with vision loss may feel uncomfortable engaging in social activities, because they are embarrassed at not being able to recognize friends and acquaintances. They may also have difficulty moving around in a crowd and in unfamiliar places, serving themselves at a buffet, or enjoying themselves without being able to see what is going on. The first step is to help your older relative get over embarrassment. As discussed in Chapter 9, explaining to friends some concerns and possible ways to handle situations that might crop up will help everyone in the long run. Practicing sighted guide techniques and familiarizing your older relative ahead of time with the environment may also help him or her overcome fears and concerns.

Some theaters and facilities now offer headsets with audio description of performances, as well as having preferred seating for people with disabilities. Audio description can make the performance quite enjoyable for someone with vision loss. Through the headset, your older relative can hear a description of the action on stage during the course of the performance like that of video description for TV programs and videos.

Similarly, at many museums your older relative can receive an audio description headset or device that describes what is on display. Most museums have improved accessibility through use of tactile displays and audio description devices through special funding for this purpose. Many also provide braille handouts, and live or recorded audio tours. You can find out about the availability of these features just by calling the museum before you visit. For individuals who enjoy art or would like to learn more, *Art Beyond Sight: A Resource Guide to Art, Creativity, and Visual Impairment* (published in 2003 by Art Education for the Blind and AFB Press) provides vital information on all aspects of exploring art and creativity by people with vision loss.

EXERCISE

Encourage your older relative to continue to exercise. According to the Centers for Disease Control and Prevention, "Every adult should accumulate 30 minutes or more of moderate physical activity over most days of the week." Of course, your relative's physician should be consulted before beginning new physical activities. Walking is a good choice. Helpful devices such as beeping balls and talking pedometers are available. If your older relative is trying out a new exercise, you may have to explain it in great detail, since he or she may not be able to see a demonstration, and offer a number of verbal cues. Sometimes people with vision loss experience balance problems; take this into account in any exercise program. Providing a sturdy chair, a steadying arm, or grab bar will help.

As you have seen in this chapter, there is no reason for your older relative to stop enjoying life just because he or she is experiencing vision loss. With a few adjustments, some training, and special equipment, leisure activities and hobbies can be just as entertaining and satisfying as they ever were. This is just as true for the more mundane, daily tasks of life as well. As you and your older relative learn new skills and different ways of going about things, you may find that you're having a good time. A sense of humor and a willingness to adapt and try new ways of doing things can make a significant difference.

Afterword

The Road Ahead

Remember Robert Mackinnon, the man whose happy ending was recounted at the beginning of this book? Were you a little dubious at first when you read about how well he adjusted to his vision loss? At this point, his story might seem quite reasonable to you, now that you know more about how people adapt to living with vision loss. Losing some of one's vision is a real challenge, but your family can make the transition successfully.

Take a moment to reread Mr. Mackinnon's story at the beginning of the introduction to this book. Is it possible for you to imagine your own family's successful adjustment to vision loss? What might it take to make that happen? What parts of this book can help you get there? Write down a brief outline of a plan if that would be helpful.

We hope that this handbook has addressed your concerns and has helped you to assist your older relative as he or she adjusts to vision loss—as well as easing any anxiety you may be feeling as you move into the adjustment process. The road ahead may have some bumps at times, but it is a busy road—thousands of other families have adjusted to vision loss successfully, and yours can, too.

Appendix

Frequently Asked Questions and Answers

As your family is adjusting to your older relative's vision loss, you'll undoubtedly have lots of questions for many different people. Although this handbook cannot possibly anticipate them all, you'll find answers to a few of the more frequently asked questions here. References to the relevant chapters and helpful resources have been included as well.

If you have additional questions, you can contact the American Foundation for the Blind (AFB). Call toll-free at (800) AFB-LINE (800-232-5463), e-mail the Information Center at afbinfo@afb.net, or visit AFB's Web site at www.afb.org. You can search for vision-related organizations and services at www.afb.org/services.asp. AFB's Web site contains valuable information on living with vision loss, information for friends and family members, vision rehabilitation services available in each state, books and resources, and many other useful items. You'll also be able to read more about AFB's National Center on Vision Loss in Dallas.

READING

My mother can't see to read any more. What should I do?

There are several solutions, depending on the type of vision loss your mother has and her current level of vision:

- If she has some usable vision, she should visit a low vision specialist who can help her with a magnification system and lighting, both of which are critical to reading. Low vision services are explained in Chapters 1 and 5. Depending on your mother's vision, adequate lighting may be all she needs.

- Many public libraries and bookstores now carry large-print books and magazines.
- She might enjoy the Talking Books program and being able to listen to books and current magazines. Talking Books are recorded materials—most often books or magazines—on audio disc and audiocassette provided by the National Library Service for the Blind and Physically Handicapped, which are available on free loan to people who are blind, visually impaired, or otherwise unable to read or use standard printed materials. To obtain Talking Books, playback equipment, and accessories, you must be registered for the Library of Congress Talking Book Program. Check the Resources section for contact information.

My mother says she can't see well enough to read. I know the lighting in her house is inadequate. Suggestions?

Proper lighting is often the key to being able to see to read. Check Chapter 7 for suggestions. Also, AFB's book *Making Life More Livable* contains many recommendations on lighting. See the Resources section for information about this book or check AFB's bookstore online at www.afb.org/store.

LEISURE ACTIVITIES

My parents used to play cards with their friends all the time. With my mother's vision loss, they feel they can no longer continue this activity. What now?

Most card games are now available in large-print and tactile (braille) versions. These are available through catalogs that specialize in vision-related products (see the Resources section for a listing of some of these catalogs). Also, there are many other games that have been adapted for people with vision loss—such as dominoes, checkers, chess, Scrabble, and Monopoly, just to mention a few.

My parents used to watch television together all the time, but now my father can't see the TV. Is there a way he can still enjoy the programs?

There are a number of possible solutions for television watching:

- One simple solution is for him to move closer to the television—or move the TV closer to his chair.
- Make sure that glare from bright light from the sun or a lamp is not shining directly on the TV screen and causing a problem for your father. You can eliminate glare by positioning the TV away from windows or using shades or mini-blinds to minimize the glare.
- Screen magnifiers that fit over the TV screen are available through the vision-related specialty catalogs listed in the Resources section. However, these provide limited magnification.
- A low vision specialist may be able to prescribe a low vision device, such as a telescope, that can help your father see the TV screen.
- Television programs and videotapes with video description of the visual elements, which is explained in Chapter 10, can make watching TV enjoyable even if your father can't see the screen.

My father can't find his favorite programs on TV anymore. He says the remote is too complicated. Does he need a special remote?

A number of different types of TV remotes are available through vision-related specialty catalogs listed in the Resources section. Some reduce the number of keys; others are available with large print, high-contrast, or tactile keys. Your father can choose which type of remote works best for him.

GETTING AROUND

My mother gets very disoriented due to her vision loss. She used to go to her outside mailbox, but she can't find it now. Will someone else have to get her mail from now on?

Your mother may be helped by an orientation and mobility (O&M) specialist who is trained to help persons with vision loss to regain their ability to get around in their home and community. Call AFB's toll-free help line (800-232-5463) or check AFB's Web directory to find services in your state and community.

I am afraid my father will fall and hurt himself, since he trips all the time. What should I do?

Often older people who are experiencing vision loss have problems with their balance, and falls are a frequent concern for their family and friends. Your dad might benefit from using a white cane, which can help both with his balance and with locating objects in his path. Again, getting help from an O&M specialist, as described in the previous answer, is a good idea. You may also want to conduct a home survey (which appears in Chapter 7) to make sure that pathways around the house are clear and that items such as throw rugs are not contributing to the problem.

When I try to walk with my aunt who has vision loss, I don't know how to help her. Is there some way to walk safely with a person who can't see?

Techniques known as "sighted guide" have been developed by vision rehabilitation professionals for sighted people walking together with people who have vision loss. Chapter 6 explains the basics of these techniques and how you can guide your aunt safely indoors and out.

My mother has fallen in her bathroom several times. She says she can't tell where things are since everything is white. What can I do to help her?

Read Chapter 7 and use the Home Survey Checklist at the end of that chapter to help you figure out how you can provide necessary color contrast in the bathroom and eliminate glare from the shiny tiles. Of course, nonskid mats and grab bars are essential to help eliminate falls in the bathroom as well.

COOKING

Cooking is a real chore for my father, although he used to enjoy it. Now he says he can't see well enough to measure ingredients, set the temperature for the stove, or even find the items in the kitchen. Does this mean he can't cook anymore?

Your father can cook again if he gets some assistance. Here are a few suggestions:

- Your father can benefit from having a vision rehabilitation therapist visit his home. Call AFB's toll-free number or check AFB's online directory for services in your area.
- Chapter 6 offers many suggestions about techniques and tools for cooking with vision loss. The vision-related specialty catalogs listed in the Resources section supply many kitchen-related aids and appliances, such as Hi-Marks for marking stove and oven settings, large-print or high-contrast measuring cups and spoons, and high-contrast cutting boards.
- Complete the Home Survey Checklist in Chapter 7 to determine some of the things you can do to make your father's kitchen easier to use.
- The book *Making Life More Livable: Simple Adaptations for Living at Home after Vision Loss* can give you additional tips on how to help your father in the kitchen and elsewhere around the house (see the Resources section).

EATING

My father is having a hard time at meals, and he absolutely refuses to go to a restaurant anymore. He says he just makes a mess at the table and can't find his food.

There are some simple techniques that can help your father get oriented to the table and find his food.

- The clock method is an excellent way to describe the location of food and items at the place setting. For example, you can tell your father that his roast beef is at noon and his water glass is at 2:00.
- Using a mat or tablecloth that contrasts with the dishes in the place setting will help him if he has some usable vision. Use of color contrast includes using drinking glasses and cups that provide contrast to the beverage that is in them.

- Put the place setting on a nonskid, contrasting surface, such as cloth or shelf liner. This material comes in different colors, can be cut to fit the situation, and is washable.
- Specialized utensils are also available from specialty catalogs, such as rocker knives, bumper guards for plates, and audible liquid level indicators so that your older relative can pour liquids safely and efficiently.

For more information about eating techniques check out Chapter 6 and the discussion of Becoming Comfortable Out in Public in Chapter 9, as well as some of the publications listed in the Resources section.

KEEPING IN TOUCH

Mom used to write me letters all the time. Now she says she can't see to write well enough. I miss her letters. Any suggestions?

As explained in Chapter 6, writing guides for letter writing, signatures, envelopes, and checks are available through vision rehabilitation agencies and through the vision-related specialty catalogs listed in the Resources section. These make it possible for people with vision loss to continue to write legibly. Your mother may need encouragement and possibly some instruction to use these.

Before losing his vision, Dad called me at least once every week. Now he says he can't read my telephone number or even dial the telephone accurately. What is the answer?

Large-print or high-contrast telephones are available through some retail stores or through the vision-related specialty catalogs listed in the Resources section. Programmable phones, in which telephone numbers can be programmed for 1- or 2-button dialing or voice dialing, are also easy to find. Some telephone companies provide directory assistance and dial phone numbers free of charge for people with visual impairments who submit their application form signed by a physician.

MANAGING MONEY

My mother can't distinguish among 1-, 5-, 10-, or 20-dollar bills when she shops. How can she avoid asking the cashier to handle her wallet and money?

Identifying and organizing money can be difficult for people when they first lose vision, but Chapter 6 provides some tips that may help, such as identifying coins by touch and folding bills in certain ways to identify them. Wallet organizers that have places to store each denomination of bill are available through catalogs that specialize in vision-related products.

BANKING

My father wants to maintain his bank account, but he can't write checks legibly anymore—much less read his statements.

There are several solutions to this problem, as explained in Chapter 6:

- Most banks can order raised-line or large-print checks for their patrons that make it easier to find the lines on which to write.
- Check-writing templates are available that make it easier to write and sign checks. These are available through local vision rehabilitation agencies or through vision-related specialty catalogs.
- Large-print check registers are also available from the same sources.
- Many banks offer online banking. This may be an option that your father may prefer if he is familiar with using a computer or is interested in doing so. (See Chapter 6 for information about screen magnification or speech output that allow people with visual impairments to use computers.) Most banks will allow you to monitor account activity over the telephone as well.

TELLING TIME

How can my father tell time, since he can't read the face of his watch anymore?

Large-numeral and talking watches are available through the vision-related specialty catalogs listed in the Resources section, as well as tactile watches on which the numbers and hands can be felt. There are many choices available to meet his needs. Low vision and talking clocks are also available.

MAINTAINING GOOD HEALTH

My father has diabetes, and now he can't see the insulin gauge to check his blood sugar or give himself shots. Is there an alternative?

There are a number of diabetic aids and appliances that can help individuals with diabetes to remain independent, such as talking glucometers for checking glucose levels and "count-a-dose" devices to ensure that insulin dosages are calibrated correctly. These devices can be found in the vision-related specialty catalogs listed in the Resources section.

My mother is on a diet and wants to be able to check her weight daily. How can she read the scale?

Talking scales are available through the vision-related specialty catalogs listed in the Resources section.

MAINTAINING YOUR APPEARANCE

My mother used to take pride in her appearance. Now she wears clothes that don't match. She lost some of her vision recently, which I believe has caused this problem. What should she do?

There are a number of methods your mother can use to distinguish her clothes. First, talk to her about the situation and tell her you will be glad to help. Stress that you want to work with her to develop a method that makes sense for her. A number of tips on how to organize clothing and drawers are offered in Chapter 7. For instance, she could place similarly colored clothes together in one section of a closet or, alternatively, hang already-matched outfits together. Books such as *Making Life More Livable*, listed in the Resources section, contain many other good ideas. Vision rehabilitation therapists will offer the most help to your mother with this and other daily tasks.

COPING AND ADJUSTMENT

My father is really having problems coping with macular degeneration. Is there any help available for him?

Your father can benefit from vision rehabilitation services, which are described in Chapter 5. He may need the help of a low vision specialist and a vision rehabilitation therapist. Older people with other types of eye conditions such as glaucoma, diabetic retinopathy, or hemianopia caused from stroke can also benefit from these services. Coping with vision loss is difficult for everyone in the beginning, but if you think your father might be having a particularly difficult time, you might want to look into a support group offered by a rehabilitation service or professional counseling. Adjustment to vision loss is discussed in Chapters 3 and 4.

MODIFYING THE ENVIRONMENT

My uncle has recently been diagnosed with visual loss. What can I do to make his home safer and easier for him to get around?

For a variety of tips for adapting the home for an older person with vision loss, read Chapter 7. You might also want to complete the Home Survey Checklist at the end of that chapter. Some general rules of thumb are as follows:
- Increase lighting.
- Eliminate glare.
- Eliminate hazards, such throw rugs.
- Create color contrast to make objects in the environment easier to see.
- Organize and label items.
- Discuss any changes in the home with your older relative so he does not become disoriented or bump into furniture that has been moved.

EMPLOYMENT

My father would like to go back to work. Is that possible with vision loss?

Believe it or not, the fastest growing segment of workers in this country consists of individuals 55 years of age and older. Your father should be encouraged to look into work options, since rehabilitation training and special equipment are available in every state for people with vision loss who want to work. Information about programs in your state can be found by contacting AFB's information center or by checking AFB's online service directory. See the Seniors section of AFB's Web site for more information on empolyment.

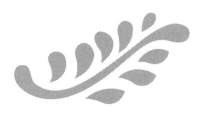

Notes

Chapter 2

1. "Diabetes Control and Complications Trial" (Bethesda, MD: National Diabetes Informational Clearinghouse, October 2001). Available online at http://diabetes.niddk.nih.gov/dm/pubs/control.

2. Lylas G. Mogk, Marja Mogk, and Carol J. Sussman-Skalka, "Charles Bonnet Syndrome," *Vision Connection* (New York: Lighthouse International). Available online at www.vision connection.org/Content/YourVision/EyeDisorders.

3. Adapted from Nora Griffin-Shirley and Gerda Groff, *Prescriptions for Independence* (New York: American Foundation for the Blind, 1993), pp. 51–57.

Chapter 3

1. Thomas J. Carroll, *Blindness: What It Is, What It Does and How to Live with It* (Boston: Little, Brown, 1961); A. Burack-Weiss, "Psychological Aspects of Aging and Vision Loss," in E. Faye, ed., *The Aging Eye and Low Vision* (New York: The Lighthouse, 1992), pp. 29–34; and Alberta. L. Orr, *Issues in Aging and Vision: A Curriculum for University Programs and In-Service Training* (New York: AFB Press, 1998).

2. Elizabeth Kübler-Ross, *On Death and Dying* (New York: Macmillan, 1969).

3. Lylas G. Mogk and Marja Mogk, *Macular Degeneration: The Complete Guide to Saving Your Sight* (New York: Ballantine Books, 2003).

4. Sam Negrin, "Psychosocial Aspects of Aging and Visual Impairment," In Randall T. Jose, ed., *Understanding Low Vision* (New York: American Foundation for the Blind, 1983), pp. 55–59.

5. L. G. Perlman, ed., *The Rehabilitation of the Older Blind Person: A Shared Responsibility,* reprint of the second Mary E. Switzer Memorial Seminar (Washington, D.C.: National Rehabilitation Association, 1977).

Chapter 4

1. T. F. DiGeronimo, *How to Talk to Your Senior Parents about Really Important Things* (San Francisco: Jossey-Bass, 2001).

2. J. P. Reinhardt and T. D'Allura, "Social Support and Adjustment to Vision Impairment across the Life Span," in B. Silverstone, M. A. Lang, B. P. Rosenthal, and E. Faye, eds., *The Lighthouse Handbook on Vision Impairment and Vision Rehabilitation, Vol. 2* (New York: Oxford University Press, 2000).

3. J. P. Reinhardt, "The Importance of Friendship and Family Support in Adaptation to Chronic Vision Impairment," *Journal of Gerontology: Psychological Sciences,* 51B (1996), pp. 268–278.

4. C. Sussman-Skalka, *Family and Friends Can Make a Difference! How to Help When Someone Close to You is Visually Impaired* (New York: Lighthouse Center for Education, 2002).

Chapter 7

1. T. F. DiGeronimo, *How to Talk to Your Senior Parents about Really Important Things* (San Francisco: Jossey-Bass, 2001), p. 13.

2. Alberta L. Orr and Priscilla Rogers, *Solutions for Success: A Training Manual for Working with Older People Who Are Visually Impaired* (New York: AFB Press, 2002); and Maureen A. Duffy, *Making Life More Livable: Simple Adaptations for Living at Home After Vision Loss* (New York: AFB Press, 2002).

3. Maureen A. Duffy, *New Independence! Environmental Adaptations in Community Facilities for Adults with Visual Impairment* (Mohegan Lake, NY: AWARE, 1997).

Chapter 8

1. H. L. Bate, "Hearing Impairment among Older Persons: A Factor in Communication," in Alberta L. Orr, ed., *Vision and Aging: Crossroads to Service Delivery* (New York: AFB Press, 1992).

Chapter 10

1. B. Bird et al., *Take Charge of Your Life* (New York: Lighthouse International, 2001).

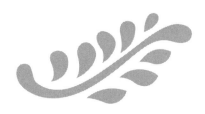

Resources

This section is designed to provide information you may need about finding a service or product that will help your older relative cope with his or her visual impairment. This resource listing provides a sample of the organizations and companies that offer assistance, information, referrals, products, and services related to vision loss and aging. If these organizations and companies do not have the answers to questions regarding older people with vision loss, they will be able to refer you to someplace that does.

For ease of use, this chapter is divided into six main sections:
- Information and referral
- Sources of vision simulators
- Products for independent living
- Resources for people with hearing impairment
- Resources for recreation
- Caregiving resources
- Further reading and information

For more complete listings of service providers, you can consult the *AFB Directory of Services for Blind and Visually Impaired Persons in the United States and Canada,* available from the American Foundation for the Blind or online at www.afb.org. You can also call AFB's Information Center at (800) AFB-LINE (232-5463).

INFORMATION AND REFERRAL

Organizations listed in this section provide general information about visual impairment and blindness, eye conditions, and adapted or specialized products and technology, as well as referrals for additional information and services.

GENERAL INFORMATION ON VISUAL IMPAIRMENT

American Academy of Ophthalmology
P.O. Box 7424
San Francisco, CA 94120-7424
(415) 561-8500
Fax: (415) 561-8533
E-mail: comm.@aao.org
www.aao.org

Professional membership association for eye care physicians that works to ensure that the public can obtain the best possible eye care. Provides information on eye health for consumers and referrals to member physicians.

American Foundation for the Blind
11 Penn Plaza, Suite 300
New York, NY 10001
(800) 232-5463 (800-AFB-LINE) or (212) 502-7600
Fax: (212) 502-7777
E-mail: afbinfo@afb.net
www.afb.org

Provides services to and acts as an information clearinghouse for people who are blind or visually impaired and their families, professionals, organizations, schools, and corporations. Has fact sheets on many aspects of visual impairment, including aging and vision loss. Stimulates research and mounts program initiatives to improve services to blind and visually impaired people. Publishes a wide variety of professional, reference, and consumer books and videos; journals; and the *AFB Directory of Services for Blind and Visually Impaired Persons in the United States and Canada.*

American Optometric Association
243 North Lindbergh Boulevard
St. Louis, MO 63141
(314) 991-4100
Fax: (314) 991-4101
www.aoanet.org

Provides information on visual conditions, eye diseases, and low vision; consumer guides for eye care; and referrals to optometrists.

Eldercare Locator
U.S. Administration on Aging
Washington, DC 20201
(800) 677-1116
www.eldercare.gov

Connects older Americans and their caregivers with sources of information on senior services and links those who need assistance with state and local area agencies on aging and community-based organizations that serve older adults and their caregivers. Eldercare Locator is a public service of the U.S. Administration on Aging.

Helen Keller National Center for Deaf-Blind Youths and Adults
141 Middle Neck Road
Sands Point, NY 11050-1218
(516) 944-8900 (Voice/TTY)
Fax: (516) 944-8637
E-mail: hkncinfo@hknc.org
www.helenkeller.org

Works to assist persons with deaf-blindness (those who have both hearing and visual impairments) in becoming as independent as possible and in enjoying a quality of life as full and productive as possible. Has an aging specialist as well.

Lighthouse International
111 East 59th Street
New York, NY 10022-1202
(800) 829-0500 or (212) 821-9200

TTD/TTY: (212) 821-9713
Fax: (212) 821-0707
E-mail: info@lighthouse.org
www.lighthouse.org
www.visionconnection.org

Works to overcome visual impairment for people of all ages
through worldwide leadership in rehabilitation services, education, research, and advocacy. Provides rehabilitation services, including training in adaptive living skills and computer skills for
seniors. Publishes the newsletter *Aging & Vision* and other publications on age-related vision loss for both professional and lay
audiences. Maintains a catalog of independent living products.

National Association for Visually Handicapped
22 West 21st Street
New York, NY 10010
(888) 205-5951 or (212) 889-3141
Fax: (212) 727-2931
E-mail: staff@navh.org
www.navh.org

3201 Balboa Street
San Francisco, CA 94121
(415) 221-3201
Fax: (415) 221-8754
E-mail: staffca@navh.org

Provides information and referral for people with low vision on
large-print books, low vision devices, medical advances and up-
dates, craft materials and projects, resource guides, and religious
materials. Sells low vision products and devices. Maintains a large-
print mail-order library. Promotes public awareness of low vision.

National Eye Care Project
Eye Care America
P.O. Box 429098
San Francisco, CA 94142-9098
(800) 222-3937 or (887) 888-6327
Fax: (415) 561-8567
www.eyecareamerica.org

Provides medical and surgical eye care for persons over 65 years of age at no out-of-pocket cost through a network of volunteer ophthalmologists around the country. Provides literature on eye diseases and procedures.

National Eye Institute
Building 31, Room 6A32
31 Center Drive, MSC 2510
Bethesda, MD 20892-2510
(301) 496-5248
Fax: (301) 402-1065
E-mail: 2020@nei.nih.gov
www.nei.nih.gov

Established by Congress in 1968 to protect and prolong the vision of the American people, NEI conducts and supports research that helps prevent and treat eye diseases and other disorders of vision. Provides information on advances in eye disease research and about clinical trials.

**National Library Service for the Blind
and Physically Handicapped**
Library of Congress
1291 Taylor Street, NW
Washington, DC 20542
(800) 424-8567 or (202) 707-5100
Fax: (202) 707-0712
TDD/TTY: (202) 707-0744
E-mail: nls@loc.gov
www.loc.gov/nls

Offers a free library service for people who are unable to read standard print materials because of a visual or physical impairment. Provides recorded Talking Books and magazines and braille publications to eligible borrowers by postage-free mail and through a network of cooperative libraries. Also distributes Talking Book machines.

**U.S. Department of Veterans Affairs
Blind Rehabilitation Service**
810 Vermont Avenue, NW

Washington, DC 20420
(888) 442-4551 or (202) 273-8481
Fax: (202) 273-7603
E-mail: wandawashington@hg.med.va.gov
www1.va.gov/blindrehab

Oversees programs for visually impaired veterans through a network of rehabilitation centers, clinics, and field staff throughout the country. Services include orientation and mobility, living skills, communication skills, activities of daily living, manual skills, computer access training, physical conditioning, recreation, adjustment to blindness, family counseling, and group meetings. Also supplies needed devices, appliances, and equipment.

SPECIFIC EYE CONDITIONS

American Diabetes Association
1701 North Beauregard Street
Alexandria, VA 22314
(800) 342-2383 or (703) 549-1500
Fax: (703) 836-7439
E-mail: customerservice@diabetes.org
www.diabetes.org

Provides information and public education about diabetes, including diabetic retinopathy, to consumers and professionals. Publishes books, journals, and brochures.

American Macular Degeneration Foundation
P.O. Box 515
Northampton, MA 01061-0515
(888) 622-8527 or (413) 268-7660
www.macular.org

Works for the prevention, treatment, and cure of macular degeneration by raising funds, educating the public, and supporting scientific research. Provides consumer information and referrals to eye care professionals.

American Society of Cataract and Refractive Surgery
4000 Legato Road, Suite 850

Fairfax, VA 22033
(703) 591-2220
Fax: (703) 591-0614
E-mail: ascrs@ascrs.org
www.ascrs.org

Provides information about cataracts and refractive surgery and referrals to ophthalmologists specializing in eye surgery.

Glaucoma Foundation
80 Maiden Lane, Suite 1206
New York, NY 10038
(800) 452-8266 or (212) 285-0080
E-mail: info@glaucomafoundation.org
www.glaucomafoundation.org

Offers information and public education about glaucoma; provides free glaucoma screenings; funds research; and publishes consumer guides and brochures and *Eye to Eye,* a quarterly newsletter.

SOURCES OF VISION SIMULATORS

The following organizations and companies distribute vision simulators, eyeglasses that simulate different types of functional vision loss. They can be used for the learning activities in this training manual. The type and cost of the simulators vary among distributors.

DAAS Consulting
P.O. Box 64164
528 B. Clarke Road
Coquitlam, BC V3J 7V6
Canada
E-mail: daascon@istar.ca

Distributes vision problem simulation kits for professionals.

Fork in the Road Vision Rehabilitation Services
5141 Door Drive
Madison, WI 53705

(608) 233-3464
E-mail: ForkintheRoad@TDS.net
www.LowVisionSimulators.com

Supplies a variety of simulators showing different degrees of various eye conditions, including age-related macular degeneration, retinitis pigmentosa, glaucoma, diabetic retinopathy, homonymous hemianopia and cataracts.

Lighthouse International
111 East 59th Street
New York, NY 10022-1202
(800) 829-0500 or (212) 821-9200
TDD/TTY: (212) 821-9713
Fax: (212) 821-9707
E-mail: info@lighthouse.org
www.lighthouse.org

Sells VisualEyes Simulators, a set of disposable eyeglasses that simulate functional vision loss.

Dr. George Zimmerman
University of Pittsburgh
School of Education
5316 Wesley Posvar Hall
Pittsburgh, PA 15260
(412) 624-7247
Fax: (412) 648-7081
www.pitt.edu/~soeforum/sped_vis.html

Sells vision simulators.

PRODUCTS FOR INDEPENDENT LIVING

SELF-HELP MATERIALS

Braille Institute of America
741 North Vermont Avenue
Los Angeles, CA 90029
(800) 272-4553 or (323) 663-1111
Fax: (323) 663-1428
E-mail: info@brailleinstitute.org
www.brailleinstitute.org

Produces and distributes *Sound Solutions,* a set of audiocassette tapes that provides independent living tips. Available free of charge to people who are visually impaired.

CIL Publications and Audiobooks
VISIONS Services for the Blind and Visually Impaired
500 Greenwich Street, 3rd floor
New York, NY 10013-1354
Fax: (212) 219-4078
(212) 625-1616
E-mail: cilpubs@visionsvcb.org
www.visionsvcb.org/cil.asp

Offers self-study audiotapes and audiobooks for people who are blind or visually impaired. Subjects include indoor mobility, personal management, and sensory development.

Hadley School for the Blind
700 Elm Street
Winnetka, IL 60093-0299
(800) 323-4238 or (847) 446-8111
Fax: (847) 446-9916
E-mail: info@hadley.edu
www.hadley.edu

Offers tuition-free distance education courses for persons who are legally blind, their family members, and professionals and paraprofessionals working in the blindness field. Courses include Conducting Self-Help Groups; You, Your Eyes, and Your Diabetes; Self-Esteem and Adjusting with Blindness; Introduction to Low Vision; Independent Living; and Recreation and Leisure Time Activities. Also offers high school courses, as well as courses in braille and communication skills, independent living, recreation and leisure, and technology.

Lighthouse International
111 East 59th Street
New York, NY 10022-1202
(800) 829-0500 or (212) 821-9200
TTD/TTY: (212) 821-9713

Fax: (212) 821-9707
E-mail: info@lighthouse.org
www.lighthouse.org

Publishes *Sharing Solutions,* an online newsletter for people with impaired vision and their support network. The newsletter includes tips for independent living and information for and about support groups. Also sells specialized products, such as adapted household products, for people with visual impairments.

CATALOGS

The companies listed in this section sell by catalog a wide variety of specialized products that help people with visual impairments and other disabilities carry out everyday activities. The types of products in each catalog are indicated in the listing.

Ableware/Maddak
661 Route 23 South
Wayne, NJ 07470
(973) 628-7600
Fax: (973) 305-0841
E-mail: custservice@maddak.com
http://service.maddak.com

Designer and manufacturer of assistive devices for activities of daily living. Offers adapted games, adapted scissors, eating utensils and tableware, enlarged grips, nonskid table mats, and writing devices.

Adaptive Solutions
1301 Azalea Road, Suite 102
P.O. Box 191087
Mobile, AL 33619-1087
(800) 299-3045 or (251) 666-3045
Fax: (251) 660-1788
www.talksight.com

Sell products such as watches, canes, and writing guides as well as aids for household, personal, and recreational use.

Ambutech
34 DeBaets Street
Winnipeg, MB R2J 3S9
Canada
(800) 561-3340 or (204) 663-3340
Fax: (800) 267-5059
E-mail: orders@ambutech.com
www.ambutech.com

Sells a wide range of mobility equipment.

American Printing House for the Blind
1839 Frankfort Avenue
P.O. Box 6085
Louisville, KY 40206-0085
(800) 223-1839 or (502) 895-2405
Fax: (502) 899-2274
E-mail: info@aph.org
www.aph.org

Distributes braille products, books, and supplies; large-print books; computer software and access products; labeling and marking products; lighting; low vision devices; mobility devices; personal care products; recreation and leisure products; talking products; and writing and reading devices.

Clotilde
P.O. Box 7500
Big Sandy, TX 75755-7500
(800) 545-4002
E-mail: customer_service@clotilde.com
www.clotilde.com

Sells sewing notions, needle threaders, and regular and adaptive sewing supplies.

Independent Living Aids
200 Robbins Lane
Jericho, NY 11753
(800) 537-2118 or (516) 937-1848
Fax: (516) 937-3906

E-mail: can-do@independentliving.com
www.independentliving.com

Distributes braille products and supplies, adapted clocks and watches, computer software and access products, diabetes management products, kitchen and housekeeping items, labeling and marking products, lighting, low vision devices, mobility devices, personal care products, recreation and leisure products, talking products, telephones and accessories, and writing and reading devices.

LS&S Group
P.O. Box 673
Northbrook, IL 60065
(800) 468-4789 or (847) 498-9777
TDD: (866) 317-8533
Fax: (847) 498-1482
E-mail: info@lssproducts.com
www.lssproducts.com

Distributes braille products and supplies, adapted clocks and watches, computer software and access products, diabetes management products, kitchen and housekeeping items, labeling and marking products, lighting, low vision devices, mobility devices, personal care products, recreation and leisure products, talking products, telephones and accessories, and writing and reading devices.

Maxi-Aids
42 Executive Boulevard
Farmingdale, NY 11735
(800) 522-6294
TTY: (800) 281-3555
Fax: (631) 752-0689
E-mail: sales@maxiaids.com
www.maxiaids.com

Distributes braille products and supplies, adapted clocks and watches, computer software and access products, diabetes management products, kitchen and housekeeping items, labeling and marking products, lighting, low vision devices, mobility devices, personal care products, recreation and leisure products, talking products, telephones and accessories, and writing and reading devices.

LIGHTING PRODUCTS

The companies listed here specialize in products that can help improve the lighting in your older relative's home or any residential setting for older persons. See also the previous section, Catalogs, for other sources of lighting, lamps, and light bulbs.

A.L.P. Lighting Components
6333 Gross Point Road
Niles, IL 60714-3915
(877) 257-5841 or (773) 774-9550
Fax: (773) 774-9331
www.alplighting.com

Manufactures a wide variety of lighting fixtures, lamps, light bulbs, louvers, reflectors, and compact fluorescent bulbs.

Dazor Manufacturing Corporation
4483 Duncan Avenue
St. Louis, MO 63110
(800) 345-9103 or (314) 652-2400
Fax: (314) 652-2069
E-mail: info@dazor.com
www.dazor.com

Manufactures a wide variety of task lights and lamps, including swing arm, combination fluorescent/incandescent, halogen, and magnifying lamps.

Philips Lighting Company
200 Franklin Square Drive
Somerset, NJ 08875-6800
(800) 555-0050
Fax: (732) 563-3740
www.lighting.philips.com

Manufactures a wide variety of light bulbs, including fluorescent, compact fluorescent, incandescent, halogen, and full spectrum.

Also provides specialty lighting and innovative lighting solutions.

PRODUCTS FOR LABELING

The companies listed here specialize in products for labeling and identification. See the Catalogs section in this appendix for other sources of products for labeling and marking, including clothing identifiers, Hi-Marks 3-D Marker, Spot 'n Line Pen, prescription labels, raised marks and dots, and marking pens and materials.

Gladys E. Loeb Foundation
2002 Forest Hill Drive
Silver Spring, MD 20903-1532
(301) 434-7748 (Voice/Fax)
E-mail: gelfdn@starpower.net

Manufactures Loeb's Labels, durable plastic nonbraille food labels in the shapes of popular fruits and vegetables, mounted on durable elastic bands.

Rx Partners Pharmacy
500 Old Pond Road, Suite 403
Bridgeville, PA 15017
(888) 477-6337
www.rxpartnerspharmacy.com

Distributor of Aloud, an audio system that reads prescription labels aloud.

Talking Prescription Labels
En-Vision America
2012 W. College Avenue
Normal, IL 61761
(800) 890-1180 or (309) 452-3088
Fax: (309) 452-3643
E-mail: envision@envisionamerica.com
www.envisionamerica.com

Distributes ScripTalk, a portable, handheld audio system that reads prescriptions aloud.

Talking Rx
P.O. Box 649
Southington, CT 06489
(888) 798-2557
www.talkingrx.com
E-mail: info@talkingrx.com

Distributes Talking Rx, an audio system that reads prescription labels aloud.

Seton Identification Products
Department AR-11
20 Thompson Road
P.O. Box 819
Branford, CT 06405-0819
(800) 571-2596
Fax: (800) 345-7819
E-mail: custsvc_setonus@seton.com
www.seton.com

Manufactures safety signs, safety labels, sign and label machines, reflective tape, warning tape, marking materials, and large-print letters.

RESOURCES FOR PEOPLE WITH HEARING IMPAIRMENT

ORGANIZATIONS AND RESOURCES

About Deafness and Hard of Hearing
http://deafness.about.com/

A resource guide to deafness/hard of hearing in the About.com web site.

Association of Late-Deafened Adults
8038 Macintosh Lane
Rockford, IL 61107
(815) 332-1515 or (866) 402-2532 (Voice/TTY)
www.alda.org

Membership organization that works with other organizations to serve the needs of late-deafened people.

Deaf Resource Center
www.deafbiz.com

Web site that lists deaf-related businesses and Web sites.

Deaf Seniors of America
Deaf Community Center
75 Bethany Road
Framingham, MA 01702
TTY: (508) 879-7658
Fax: (508) 879-7651
E-mail: dsa@deafseniors.org
www.deafseniors.org

Membership organization for people aged 50 and older who are deaf. Holds conferences and publishes newsletters and other communications for its members.

Helen Keller National Center for Deaf-Blind Youths and Adults

See listing under Information and Referral.

National Association of the Deaf
8630 Fenton Street, Suite 820
Silver Spring, MD 20910-3876
(301) 587-1788
TDD: (301) 587-1789
Fax: (301) 587-1791
E-mail: nadinfo@nad.org
www.nad.org

Membership organization that advocates to promote, protect, and preserve the rights and quality of the life of people who are deaf and hard of hearing in the United States.

Self Help for Hard of Hearing People
7910 Woodmont Avenue, Suite 1200
Bethesda, Maryland 20814
(301) 657-2248
TDD: (301) 657-2249
Fax: (301) 913-9413

E-mail: info@hearingloss.org
www.hearingloss.org

Offers educational materials and information about hearing loss and advocates for people with hearing loss.

VENDORS OF AIDS AND DEVICES FOR PEOPLE WHO ARE DEAF OR HARD OF HEARING

Harris Communications
15155 Technology Drive
Eden Prairie, MN 55344
(800) 825-6758 or (952) 906-1180
TTY: (800) 825-9187 or (952) 906-1198
E-mail: info@harriscomm.com
www.harriscomm.com

Hitec International
8160 Madison Avenue
Burr Ridge, IL 60527
(800) 288-8303 or (630) 654-9200
TDD: (800) 536-8890
Fax: (888) 654-9219
E-mail: info@hitec.com
www.hitec.com

Independent Living Aids
200 Robbins Lane
Jericho, NY 11753
(800) 537-2118 or (516) 937-1848
Fax: (516) 937-3906
E-mail: can-do@independentliving.com
www.independentliving.com

Lighthouse International
111 East 59th Street
New York, NY 10022-1202
(800) 829-0500 or (212) 821-9200
Fax: (212) 821-9707

TDD/TTY: (212) 821-9713
E-mail: info@lighthouse.org
www.lighthouse.org

LS&S Group
P.O. Box 673
Northbrook, IL 60065
TTY: (866) 317-8533
Fax: (877) 498-1482
E-mail: info@lssproducts.com
www.lssproducts.com

MaxiAids
42 Executive Boulevard
Farmingdale, NY 11735
(800) 522-6294
TTY: (800) 281-3555
Fax: (631) 752-0689
E-mail: sales@maxiaids.com
www.maxiaids.com

Potomac Technology
One Church Street, Suite 101
Rockville, MD 20850-4158
(800) 433-2838 (Voice/TTY)
Fax: (301) 762-1892
www.potomactech.com

RESOURCES FOR RECREATION

READING

The sources listed here provide reading materials in alternate formats, including large-print, braille, or audio formats. See also the Products for Independent Living section in this appendix for products that can help with reading, such as closed-circuit television systems, computer adaptations, computer hardware and software, and additional large-print reading materials, including cookbooks. For further reading resources including electronic texts, consult National Library Service Factsheets.

Betty Crocker
P.O. Box 9452
Minneapolis, MN 55440
(800) 446-1898
Fax: (763) 764-8330

Offers popular recipes using Betty Crocker products. The Betty Crocker cookbook is available on computer disk for $35.00. Recipes in large print on 9" × 12" cards are free.

Books Aloud
150 E. San Fernando Street
San Jose, CA 95112-3580
(408) 808-2613
Fax: (408) 808-4625
E-mail: info@booksaloud.org
www.booksaloud.org

Offers "Reading by Listening" program, which provides a wide variety of recorded reading material free of charge to eligible individuals.

Choice Magazine Listening
85 Channel Drive
Port Washington, NY 11050
(888) 724-6423 or (516) 883-8280
Fax: (516) 944-6849
E-mail: choicemag@aol.com
www.choicemagazinelistening.org

A free monthly anthology of current articles chosen from over 100 leading magazines recorded in four-track Library of Congress format. Distributed free through regional libraries. Also available through individual subscription.

Doubleday Large Print Home Library
1225 South Market Street
Mechanicsburg, PA 17055

E-mail: service@doubledaylargeprint.com
www.doubledaylargeprint.com

Offers a large-print Book-of-the-Month Club.

Guideposts
39 Seminary Hill Road
Carmel, NY 10512
(800) 932-2145
Fax: (845) 228-2151

True first-person stories by everyday people and well-known celebrities. Published monthly in large print.

Hansen House Music
Golden Music Big Note Songs
1820 West Avenue
Miami Beach, FL 33139
(305) 532-5461
Fax: (305) 672-8729
E-mail: info@hansenhousemusic.com
www.hansenhousemusic.com

Sells a wide selection of music books. Music notes are ½ inch across with the name of the note written inside the note. A free catalog is available.

Matilda Ziegler Magazine for the Blind
80 Eighth Avenue, Room 1304
New York, NY 10011
(212) 242-0263
Fax: (212) 633-1601
E-mail: blind@verizon.net
www.zieglermag.org

Free monthly general-interest periodical published in braille and on audiocassette.

National Library Service for the Blind
and Physically Handicapped
Library of Congress
1291 Taylor Street, NW

Washington, DC 20542
(800) 424-8567 or (202) 707-5100
TDD/TTY: (202) 707-0744
Fax: (202) 707-0712
E-mail: nls@loc.gov
www.loc.gov/nls

Provides a free library service for people who are unable to read standard print materials because of a visual or physical impairment. Recorded Talking Books and magazines and braille publications are delivered to eligible borrowers by postage-free mail and through a network of cooperative libraries. Also distributes Talking Book machines. Local libraries often have applications for this service as well. Also check with the vision rehabilitation agency in your area.

New York Times Large-Type Weekly
609 Greenwich Street, 6th Floor
New York, NY 10014
(800) 631-2580 or (212) 905-3391
Fax: (212) 905-3436
E-mail: barber@nytimes.com
http://nytimes.com

Publishes a weekly news summary from the *New York Times* in 16-point print.

Reader's Digest Partners for Sight Foundation
Reader's Digest Road
Pleasantville, NY 10570
E-mail: PartnersForSight@rd.com
www.rd.com/partnersforsight/index.jsp

Publishes *Reader's Digest Large Print for Easier Reading*.

ELECTRONIC TEXTS

This listing provides a sample of Web sites that offer books and other texts in a wide variety of electronic formats. Some are available free of charge; others have a variety of payment options. For a comprehensive list of electronic text resources, con-

tact the National Library Service or see their fact sheet at http://
lcweb.loc.gov/nls/reference/factsheets/etexts.html.

Accessible Book Collection
www.accessiblebookcollection.org
(703) 631-1585
Fax: (775) 256-2556
E-mail: customerservice@accessiblebookcollection.org

Audible.com
www.audible.com
(973) 837-2845
(888) 283-5051

Bartleby.com.
www.bartleby.com
E-mail: bartlebycom@aol.com

Bookshare.org
www.bookshare.org/web/Welcome.html
(650) 475-5440
E-mail: info@bookshare.org

ClassicReader.com
www.classicreader.com

eBooks.com
http://usa2.ebooks.com

Electronic Text Center
http://etext.lib.virginia.edu
(434) 924-3230
E-mail: etextcenter@virginia.edu

Fictionwise
www.fictionwise.com
(973) 701-6771

4Literature
www.4literature.net
E-mail: jaret.wilson@javatar.net

netLibrary
www.netlibrary.com
(800) 413-4557
E-mail: sales@netlibrary.com

The Online Books Page
www.onlinebooks.library.upenn.edu/
(215) 898-7091
E-mail: onlinebooks@pobox.upenn.edu

Page by Page Books
www.pagebypagebooks.com
E-mail: contact@PagebyPageBooks.com

Project Gutenberg
www.gutenberg.org

Tiflolibros: E-Books for the Blind
www.tiflolibros.com.ar
tiflolibros@tiflolibros.com.ar

Tumble Readables: Online Large-Print Library
www.tumblebooks.com/tumblereadable/default.asp
(416) 781-4010
Fax: (416) 781-2764
E-mail (general information): info@tumblebooks.com
E-mail (orders): orders@tumblebooks.com

RADIO READING SERVICES

International Association of Audio Information Services
WVTF Public Radio
4235 Electric Road, Suite 105

Roanoke, VA 24014
(800) 280-5325
Fax: (504) 776-2727
www.iaais.org

International organization of radio reading services, which provide audio access to information for people who are print disabled (blind, visually impaired, learning disabled, or physically disabled), including news, feature stories, sports, advertisements, and other special programs. Connects listeners with services in their area.

InTouch Networks
15 West 65th Street
New York, NY 10023
(212) 769-6270
Fax: (212) 769-6270
E-mail: intouchinfo@jgb.org
http://66.40.142.226/InTouch/default.asp

Provides national programming services for local radio reading services for people who are blind or visually impaired. Offers closed-circuit radio broadcasts of national and local newspapers and magazines.

VIDEO DESCRIPTION

Some television programs and films on videotape are available in video-described versions in which explanations and descriptions of the visual elements are inserted on the sound track without interfering with the sounds and dialogue that are part of the program. For some television programs, these descriptions can be heard on a Secondary Audio Program (SAP), a separate audio channel available on most stereo televisions sold in the United States. Programs are available on many public broadcasting and cable stations, and video described movies can be purchased or borrowed from some libraries and video stores.

Descriptive Video Service
Media Access Group at WGBH
125 Western Avenue
Boston, MA 02134

(617) 300-3600 (Voice/TDD)
(800) 333-1203 (Pre-recorded information line)
Fax: (617) 300-1020
E-mail: access@wgbh.org
www.wgbh.org/access

Narrative Television Network
5840 South Memorial Drive, Suite 312
Tulsa, OK 74145
(918) 627-1000
Fax: (918) 627-4101
E-mail: narrative@aol.com
www.narrativeTV.com

OTHER RECREATIONAL OPPORTUNITIES

The organizations listed here provide information on just two of the many recreational opportunities available to people who are blind or visually impaired.

American Blind Bowlers Association
c/o Wilbert Turner, President
3041 E. 121st Street
Cleveland, OH 44129
(216) 561-6864
E-mail: abbasecretary@earthlink.net
www.americanblindbowlers.com

Promotes bowling for people who are blind or visually impaired.

United States Blind Golf Association
3094 Shamrock Street North
Tallahassee, FL 32309
(850) 893-4511
E-mail: pomod@charter.net
www.blindgolf.com

Provides opportunities for golfers who are blind or visually impaired to compete with their peers.

CAREGIVING RESOURCES

Children of Aging Parents
P.O. Box 167
Richboro, PA 18954
(800) 227-7294
www.caps4caregivers.org

Offers caregivers of aging parents information and advice on caregiving. Has outreach programs through new support groups, workshops, and presentations for churches, schools, employers, service clubs, and television audiences.

Family Caregiver Alliance (FCA)
180 Montgomery Street, Suite 1100
San Francisco, CA 94104
www.caregiver.org
(800) 445-8106 or (415) 434-3388

Offers programs at national, state, and local levels to support and sustain caregivers. Established the National Center on Caregiving to advance the development of high-quality, cost-effective programs and policies for caregivers in every state in the country.

National Alliance for Caregiving
4720 Montgomery Lane, 5th Floor
Bethesda, MD 20814
www.caregiving.org
E-mail: info@caregiving.org

Coalition of national organizations focusing on issues of family caregiving. Conducts research, does policy analysis, develops national programs, and increases public awareness of family caregiving issues.

National Association of Professional Geriatric Care Managers
1604 N. Country Club Road
Tucson, AZ 85716-3102
(520) 881-8008
Fax: (520) 325-7925
www.caremanager.org

Nonprofit association of professional practitioners whose purpose is the development, advancement, and promotion of humane and dignified social, psychological, and health care for the elderly and their families through counseling, treatment, and the delivery of concrete services by qualified, certified providers. A list of professional care managers, by zip code, from the membership can be obtained from the Web site.

National Family Caregivers Association
10400 Connecticut Avenue, Suite 500
Kensington, MD 20895-3944
(800) 896-3650 or (301) 942-6430
Fax: (301) 942-2302
E-mail: info@thefamilycaregiver.org
www.nfcacares.org

Supports, empowers, educates, and advocates for caregivers of chronically ill, aged, or disabled family members.

Well Spouse Foundation
63 W. Main Street, Suite H
Freehold, NJ 07728
www.wellspouse.org

National membership organization that provides support to wives, husbands, and partners of the chronically ill or disabled individuals.

FURTHER READING AND INFORMATION

The following books and videos are available from AFB Press through American Foundation for the Blind's Web site at www.afb.org/store or by contacting AFB Press at (800) 232-3044 or at afborder@abdintl.com. Most books are available on cassette or ASCII disk, as well as in print.

BOOKS

AFB Directory of Services for Blind and Visually Impaired Persons in the United States and Canada, 27th edition (2005)
A comprehensive directory of information on blindness and

visual impairment, including more than 1,500 organizations, agencies, and product manufacturers, with state-by-state and province-by-province listings of organizations; descriptions of services, legislation, and key agencies in the blindness field.

Diversity and Visual Impairment: The Influence of Race, Gender, Religion, and Ethnicity on the Individual, edited by Jane Erin and Madeline Milian (2001)
An exploration of how cultural, social, and religious factors play an important role in the way an individual perceives and copes with a visual impairment. Examines how members of specific groups regard and deal with visual impairment and how their perspectives can affect their self-esteem and social relationships, as well as service delivery by professionals.

Issues in Aging and Vision: A Curriculum for University Programs and In-Service Training, by Alberta L. Orr (1998)
A curriculum addressing vision loss and its correlation with aging, covering key issues from the physical to the psychosocial.

Making Life More Livable: Simple Adaptations for Living at Home after Vision Loss, revised by Maureen A. Duffy (2002)
A guide for adults experiencing vision loss and their family and friends. Includes practical tips with numerous photographs that show how people who are visually impaired can continue living independent, productive lives at home on their own. Useful general guidelines and room-by-room specifics provide simple and effective solutions for making homes accessible and everyday activities doable for individuals with visual impairments.

Out of the Corner of My Eye: Living with Vision Loss in Later Life, by Nicolette Pernot Ringgold (1991)
A down-to-earth, upbeat, personal account about living with macular degeneration told from the perspective of an 87-year-old retired college teacher.

Prescriptions for Independence: Working with Older People Who Are Visually Impaired, by Nora Griffin-Shirley and Gerda Groff (1983)

A guide for service providers that offers helpful tips and techniques for helping elderly individuals maintain greater independence.

Self-Advocacy Skills Training for Older Individuals: Training Manual, Participant Manual, Family Guide to Self-Advocacy, by Alberta L. Orr and Priscilla Rogers (2003)
A training kit, which includes a guide for group leaders conducting self-advocacy skills training; a user-friendly manual for older group participants; and a handy, helpful booklet for family members in several accessible formats. Ideal for use in support group sessions, workshops, and training sessions.

Solutions for Success: A Training Manual for Working with Older People Who Are Visually Impaired, by Alberta L. Orr and Priscilla Rogers (2002)
A curriculum for caregivers that provides information and techniques in 20 easy-to-follow lessons, each dealing with a different aspect of visual impairment and daily living, including bathing, dressing, eating, walking, shopping, and attending to personal business.

Vision and Aging: Crossroads for Service Delivery, edited by Alberta L. Orr (1992)
A discussion of the vital services needed to address the needs of elderly persons with visual impairments for individuals working with the elderly population in any service capacity.

Vision Loss in an Aging Society: A Multidisciplinary Perspective, edited by John E. Crews and Frank J. Whittington (2000)
An analysis of the practical and public policy issues related to aging and visual impairment for people who teach or work in the fields of low vision, social work, geriatric medicine, or other areas of public health.

VIDEOS

Aging and Vision: Declaration of Independence (1984)
Five profiles of individuals who have successfully coped with visual impairment in their later years. Offers practical suggestions on how to live independent, active, and satisfying lives.

Blindness: A Family Matter (1986)
An examination of the effects of visual impairment on family members through the experiences of actual families.

Profiles in Aging and Vision, by Alberta L. Orr (1998)
An overview of the vision-related services available to older, visually impaired individuals, illustrated with interviews and personal accounts.

Solutions for Everyday Living for Older People with Visual Impairments, by Alberta L. Orr and Priscilla Rogers (2002)
A companion video to the *Solutions for Success* curriculum that presents a positive and helpful view of how older people who have lost some or all of their vision can continue to lead satisfying lives within supportive environments.

What Do You Do When You See a Blind Person? (2000)
Illustrates the simple ways to provide assistance, if needed, to someone who is blind or visually impaired and offers a fresh perspective to how to interact comfortably with someone who is visually impaired.

BROCHURES

Aging and Vision: Making the Most of Impaired Vision (1987)
Informative pamphlet on helping individuals who are elderly cope with visual impairment in real, practical ways. Offers helpful tips for improving lighting, decorating with contrasting colors, and using devices for independent living.

Consider Older Workers Who Are Visually Impaired
A brochure that explains positive reasons to hire older persons with visual impairments for employers as well as reasonable accommodations that make this feasible.

PUBLICATIONS FROM OTHER SOURCES

Family and Friends Can Make a Difference! How to Help When Someone Close to You is Visually Impaired, by C. Sussman-Skalka, (New York: Lighthouse Center for Education, 2002).

How to Talk to Your Senior Parents about Really Important Things, by T. F. DiGeronimo (San Francisco: Jossey-Bass, 2001).

Macular Degeneration: The Complete Guide to Saving Your Sight, by L. Mogk and M. Mogk (New York: Ballantine Books, 2003).

Index

About the Authors

Alberta L. Orr, MSW, is Program Manager, Aging and Vision Loss, American Foundation for the Blind (AFB) in New York City, as well as former Director of AFB's National Aging Program. She is also an adjunct faculty member at Hunter College of the City University of New York (CUNY), where she teaches Rehabilitation Counseling with the Aged in the masters' level Vision Rehabilitation program. She is also a Ph.D. candidate in social welfare at the CUNY Graduate Center.

Ms. Orr is the author or co-author of numerous publications, including *Vision and Aging: Crossroads for Service Delivery; Issues in Aging and Vision: A Curriculum for University Programs and In-Service Training, Solutions for Success: A Training Manual for Working with Older People Who are Visually Impaired;* and *Self-Advocacy Skills Training for Older Individuals Who Are Visually Impaired;* as well as the executive producer of the video, *Profiles in Aging and Vision* and co-producer of *Solutions for Everyday Living for Older People with Visual Impairments.* An internationally and nationally recognized speaker in the area of aging and vision loss. she spearheaded the National Agenda on Vision and Aging and was the convener of the National Aging and Vision Network, initiatives supported by AFB, and was twice a delegate to the White House Conference on Aging.

Her primary areas of interest are developing training materials on aging and vision loss for professionals outside the vision field and ensuring that family members have the resources they need to assist their older relatives who are experiencing vision loss to achieve maximum personal independence.

Priscilla Rogers, Ph.D., is a consultant in vision and aging with the American Foundation for the Blind (AFB) in Morristown, Tennessee. Her background includes a degree in gerontology and in special education with an emphasis in vision and aging. She is former director of the Adjustment Training Program for Older Blind at the Tampa Lighthouse for the Blind; director of Channel Markers for the Blind (now the Watson Center); Bureau Chief of Client Services for the Florida Division of Blind Services; and Commissioner of the Department for the Blind in Kentucky.

Dr. Rogers has authored several articles on vision and aging and was co-author of *A Training Manual for Working with Older People Who are Visually Impaired;* and *Self-Advocacy Skills Training for Older Individuals Who Are visually Impaired,* as well as co-producer of the video *Solutions for Everyday Living for Older People with Visual Impairments.*

In working directly with older people with vision loss and their family members, Dr. Rogers realized early on the need that family members have for information about how to help their spouse or parent cope with vision loss. Throughout her career she has advocated for the inclusion of services to family members as part of vision rehabilitation programs. The needs of family members remains a primary focus for her as vision and aging consultant with AFB, where she has conducted family training courses and focus groups with family members.